# Dictionary of Psychiatry

Edited by
Harold Thakurdas, MA (Psych), BSc, MB, BS, DPM,
and Dip. Journalism
Lyn Thakurdas, BA (Hons), Oxon

Revised by
Betty Thakurdas, SRN, SCM, Cert. Child Psych.

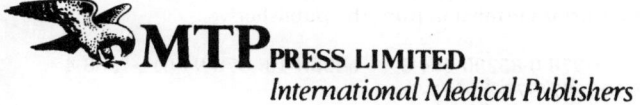
**MTP** PRESS LIMITED
*International Medical Publishers*

Published by
MTP Press Limited
Falcon House
Lancaster, England

ISBN-13: 978-0-85200-264-3     e-ISBN-13: 978-94-011-7888-4
DOI: 10.1007/978-94-011-7888-4

# Introductory Note

I have enjoyed the privilege of revising the manuscript for this dictionary whilst at the same time being the wife of one of the editors and the mother of the other.

New terms are frequently necessitated by recent advances in psychiatry and allied subjects like endocrinology, neurology, physiology, psychology, sociology and statistics, and in addition sub-specialities like child, forensic, mental handicap, psychosomatic and psychosexual disorders.

The dictionary has been designed as a ready reference for doctors taking diplomas or membership examinations in psychiatry, medical students, all grades of psychiatric nurses, social workers, administrative staff or anybody involved with psychiatric patients in the hospital or out in the community. A major work like the *International Encyclopaedia of Social Services* should be consulted for a detailed reference, e.g. on a sociological word such as 'caste'.

Drug therapy has on purpose been omitted. A number of appendices have been included, e.g. Appendix A provides the latest International Classification of Mental Disorders and Appendix F an *aide-mémoire* of essential statistical formulae.

BETTY THAKURDAS

July 1978
Lancaster,
England

## ACKNOWLEDGMENTS

1 Mental Health Act, 1959. HMSO, London

2 Mental Health (Amendment) Act, 1975. HMSO, London

3 Mental Health Act, 1959. A review by the Medical Protection Society, 1967. 50 Hallam Street, London W1N 6DE

4 *A Glossary of Mental Disorders*, 1968. HMSO, London

## REFERENCES

1 *Encyclopaedia of Psychiatry*, edited by Denis Leigh, C. M. B. Pare and John Marks, 1972. Roche Products Ltd, London

2 *A Guide to Psychiatric and Psychological Terminology*, 1962. Out of print

# Contents

# Contents

# A

**Abasia**   Inability to walk.

**Aberration**   Deviation from the normal.

**Abdominal reflexes**   Contraction of the muscles of the anterior abdominal wall when the skin of the abdomen is scratched. (Th 8 to 12.)

**Abducens nerve**   Sixth, motor nerve supplies the lateral rectus muscle of the eye.

**Abient**   Negatively oriented response.

**Ability**   Power to perform physical or mental act.

**Abortion**   Termination of pregnancy.

**Abreaction**   Release of pent-up emotions by hypnosis, intravenous injection of barbiturates or methedrine, and inhalation of ether or carbon dioxide.

**Absence**   1 Loss of consciousness in an hysterical attack; 2 petit mal.

**Abstinence syndrome**   Withdrawal syndrome.

**Abstract thinking**   Ability to use concepts and ideas independently of concrete objects.

**Abulia**   Absence of will-power or wish-power.

**Acalculia**   Loss of ability to calculate.

**Accessible**   When a psychiatrist makes a rapport with a patient; and inaccessible if he fails.

**Accident proneness**   Tendency to accidents.

**Acculturation**   Acquiring of a culture through contact.

**Acting out**   Reduction of emotional distress by the release of disturbed behaviour, which is unconsciously determined and reflects previous unresolved conflicts and attitudes.

**Action**   Purposeful behaviour.

**Actus reus**   Guilty act.

**Acute**    Illness rapid in onset and of short duration, in contrast to subacute or chronic.

**Addiction**    True dependence on drugs (as opposed to habituation) has four characteristics: 1 craving for the drug; 2 increasing tolerance for it; 3 psychological and physiological dependence on it; and 4 harmful effects on the individual and the society, e.g. alcohol and opium. (*Cf.* drug dependence; habituation.)

**Adiadochokinesis**    Loss of power to perform rapid alternating movements.

**Adient**    Positively oriented response.

**Adlerian**    Approach developed by Alfred Adler (1870–1937), who founded his own movement of individual psychology in 1911 with emphasis on the struggle for power and social factors. His groups were called Adlerian groups.

**Adolescence**    Period between puberty and adulthood ranging from 11 to 19 years, called 'teenage'; and divided into early and late adolescence.

**Aerophagy**    Swallowing of air.

**Aetiology**    Causes of disease.

**Affect**    Emotion, feeling or mood. Disorder of affect may occur in various psychiatric illnesses.

**Affective disorders**    Group of psychoses with morbid changes of mood of either depression or mania which recur and remit.

**Affiliative**    Term used in connection with communication referring to peer level as distinct from hierarchical interaction.

**Ageusia**    Absence of sense of taste.

**Aggression**    Responses intended to injure or damage a vulnerable object. Occurs in drug dependence, dementia, epilepsy, hypomania and mania, psychopathic personality and schizophrenia.

**Agnosia**   Loss of ability to recognize various stimuli, such as visual, auditory and tactile.

**Agraphia**   Loss of ability to write.

**Air-encephalography**   The X-raying of the ventricles and subarachnoid spaces after introduction of air by lumbar or cisternal puncture. Also known as pneumoencephalography.

**Akathisia**   Motor restlessness.

**Alalia**   Loss of ability to talk.

**Alcoholics Anonymous**   Organization run by ex-alcoholics for the rehabilitation of alcoholics. (AA)

**Alcoholism**   Dependence on alcohol resulting in psychological and/or physiological impairment. Bogen (1932) gives an approximate correlation of the amount of alcohol present in blood and the mental state:

Less than 1 mg per ml of blood .   .  .   .   dry and decent
1–2 mg .  .  .  .  .  .  .  .  . delighted and devilish
2–3 mg .  .  .  .  .  .  . delinquent and disgusting
3–4 mg .  .  .  .  .  .  .  .  .. dizzy and delirious
4–5 mg .  .  .  .  .  .  .  . dazed and dejected
5 mg and over .  .  .  .  .  .  .  . dead drunk

**Alexia**   Loss of ability to read; word blindness.

**Altruism**   Principle of living and acting for the sake of others.

**Alzheimer's disease**   Presenile dementia associated with cortical cerebral atrophy.

**Amaurotic family idiocy**   Mental deficiency with paralysis and blindness; and a characteristic cherry-red spot on the macula. (*Syn.* Tay-Sach's disease.)

**Ambivalence**   Contradictory emotional feelings towards an object, e.g. love and hate for a person. It is normal in interpersonal relationships, but when it occurs to a marked degree it is morbid.

**Ambiversion**  Balance of the traits between introversion and extraversion.

**Amenorrhoea**  Absence of menstruation.

**Amentia**  Arrested development of the mind from birth in contrast to the acquired condition of dementia in later life. (*Syn.* mental subnormality or deficiency.)

**Amnesia**  Loss of memory. May be partial or complete; and recent or remote, e.g. memory for recent events is lost in organic brain disease.

**Amok**  Going berserk

**Amusia**  Inability to recognize or reproduce melodies due to brain lesion.

**Anaclitic**  Emotional dependence on others; lean against; support.

**Anaesthesia**  Inability to feel touch.

**Analgesia**  Inability to feel pain.

**Analysand**  Individual being psychoanalysed.

**Analytical psychology**  School of psychology developed by Carl Gustav Jung. (*Cf.* Jungian.)

**Anamnesis**  Medical term for the history of an illness as given by the patient.

**Anankastic personality**  Essential trait is rigidity, perfectionism and meticulousness. (*Syn.* obsessional personality.)

**Anarthria**  Inability to pronounce words.

**Anergia**  Loss of energy; weakness.

**Aneurysm**  Weak bulge in an arterial wall.

**Angioma**  Collection of abnormal arteries, capillaries and veins.

**Anima**  Jungian term describing the unconscious female image in men; and animus, the unconscious male image in women.

**Ankle jerk** Foot is dorsiflexed in order to put the tendo Achilles on the stretch. A tap on the posterior surface results in a sharp contraction of the calf muscles. (S 1, S 2.)

**Anolingus** Apposition of tongue to the rectum.

**Anomaly** Marked deviation from normal.

**Anorexia** Loss of appetite.

**Anorexia nervosa** Loss of appetite in young persons of hysterical disposition.

**Anosmia** Loss of sense of smell.

**Anoxia** Lack of oxygen which may cause damage to tissues. The brain is particularly susceptible to anoxia.

**Anterior horns** Part of spinal grey matter containing motor nerve cells.

**Anterograde amnesia** Failure to recall events occurring after the onset of amnesia.

**Anthropology** Scientific study of man, his origins, development and place in social organizations.

**Antisocial personality** Individual who offends against society, having abnormally aggressive and seriously irresponsible conduct.

**Anxiety** Emotional disorder characterized by uncertainty, apprehensiveness and unresolved fear. Anxiety is the Alpha and Omega of psychiatry. It is a fear response, e.g. fight or flight. Also known as anxiety state, anxiety reaction and anxiety neurosis.

**Apathy** Attitude of indifference.

**Aphasia** Loss of ability to express meaning by the use of speech or writing, or understand spoken or written language; the former being described as motor and the latter as sensory aphasia.

**Aphonia**  Inability to phonate normally despite normal articulation, with the result that subject talks in a whisper. Often a hysterical symptom.

**Aphrodisiac**  Substance which excites sexual desire.

**Apoplexy**  Cerebral haemorrhage or thrombosis, usually causing loss of consciousness; stroke.

**Apperception**  Process of interpreting, recognizing or identifying a perception.

**Aptitude**  Ability to acquire skill of specialized nature; potential ability.

**Arachnoid mater**  The web-like middle layer of the meninges.

**Argyll–Robertson pupil**  An irregular pupil reacting to accommodation but not to light $(A + R -)$.

**Arousal**  State of cortical excitation.

**Arteriography**  The X-raying of the blood vessels after injecting an artery with opaque dye.

**Arteriosclerotic psychosis**  Acute or chronic brain syndrome due to cerebrovascular disease.

**Assault and battery**  Assault is an unlawful display of force. Battery is the intentional use of unlawful force.

**Astasia**  Inability to stand when there is no organic lesion.

**Astasia-abasia**  Inability to stand or walk in the absence of an organic lesion. Found in conversion hysteria.

**Asthenia**  Lack of vitality; weakness.

**Asylum**  'Place safe from violence or pillage'; now psychiatric hospital.

**Ataxia**  Loss or impairment of muscular co-ordination, resulting in an inability to perform accurate voluntary movement.

**Athetosis**  Slow writhing involuntary movements.

**Athletic physique**  Kretschmer's strong and muscular type.

**Attitude**   Predisposition to react positively or negatively to some degree toward an object, institution or class of persons.

**Auditory nerve**   Eighth, sensory nerve consists of two parts: the cochlear and the vestibular. Also known as acoustic nerve.

**Aura**   Warning symptoms of an attack of epilepsy or migraine.

**Autism**   Features of childhood psychosis or autism are: 1 gross and sustained impairment of emotional relationships with people; 2 apparent unawareness of personal identity to a degree inappropriate to the child's age; 3 pathological pre-occupation with particular objects; 4 sustained obsessional resistance to environmental changes; 5 abnormal perceptual experiences (in the absence of obvious organic abnormality); 6 acute, excessive and seemingly illogical anxiety; 7 serious intellectual retardation with surviving islets of normal, near normal or exceptional intellectual function; 8 mobility disturbances, hyperkinesis, queer postures, rocking; and 9 failure to acquire, loss or disturbance of speech.

**Autistic**   Behaviour controlled by factors within the individual rather than by the reality situation.

**Autistic thinking**   Mental activity controlled exclusively by the thinker.

**Autochthonous ideas**   Delusional ideas which come into the mind independently of the train of thought and alien to the normal mode of thought. This is typical of schizophrenia.

**Automatic obedience**   When an individual strictly obeys a command.

**Automatism**   No act is punishable if it is done involuntarily. In case of non-insane automatism the accused bears the burden of adducing evidence; and in case of insane automatism the accused bears the additional burden of proof.

**Autonomic**   Part of the nervous system which is concerned with the constant regulation of body functions which are not under the conscious control of the individual. The autonomic nervous system is sub-divided into sympathetic and parasympathetic.

**Autosomes**   Chromosomes other than the sex chromosomes.

**Auto-suggestion**   Suggestion arising from the individual himself.

**Aversion therapy**   Vomiting induced in alcoholism by apomorphine injection or painful electric shocks in sexual perversions.

**Aversive stimulus**   Noxious stimulus, e.g. an electric shock.

**Axon**   Longest process of a nerve cell.

# B

**Babinski reflex**   Extension of the great toe on scratching the sole.

**Backwardness**   Educational retardation due to extrinsic causes.

**Battered baby syndrome**   Collection of signs and symptoms occurring in children who have suffered repeated injuries at the hands of their parents and others.

**Battered wife syndrome**   Woman who has suffered serious or repeated physical injury from the man with whom she lives. (*Opp.* battered husband syndrome.)

**Behaviour**   Change or response of any entity or system in relation to its environment. Fore-runner of modern stimulus–response (S–R) psychology.

**Behaviourism**   School of psychology concerned with observable responses in subjects, rather than with other internal processes. It stresses objectivity.

**Behaviour therapy**   Principles of learning theories applied to the treatment of psychiatric disorders, also called behaviour modification and conditioning therapy.

**Belle indifférence**   Bland indifference in spite of distressing complaints. Occurs in hysteria.

**Bell's mania**   Acute manic excitement.

**Bell's palsy**   Paralysis of one side of the face.

**Bender visual-motor Gestalt test**   Test for ability. Consists of designs to be copied.

**Bene–Anthony family relations test**   Projective personality test. Assesses child's relationships within the family.

**Benton revised visual retention test**   Test for brain damage which relies on the patient's ability to use visual memory effectively.

**Bestiality**   Sexual relationships with animals.

**Biceps jerk**   Elbow is flexed to a right-angle and the forearm placed in a semipronated position. A tap on the thumb placed on the biceps tendon contracts the biceps. (C 5, C 6.)

**Bigamy**   Whoever, being married, marries any other person during the life of the former husband or wife is guilty of bigamy, punishable by seven years' imprisonment.

**Binovular twins**   Twins developed from two ova with different genetic make up.

**Bitemporal hemianopia**   Loss of the outer halves of both fields of vision.

**Blocking**   Sudden stoppage in the train of thought.

**Borderline**   Mental state on the boundary between neurosis and psychosis.

**Boredom**   Lethargy produced by monotony or disinterest.

**Bradyphrenia**   Retardation of mental processes.

**Broca's area**   Motor speech area situated in the left frontal lobe of the brain in right-handed person.

**Brown–Séquard syndrome** Signs produced by damage to one half of the spinal cord.

**Brushfield spots** Fine white speckling of the iris in Trisomy 21 (Down's syndrome).

**Buffoonery syndrome** Grotesque grimaces and gestures seen in catatonic schizophrenia and Ganser syndrome.

**Bulbar** Concerning the medulla oblongata.

**Burr-hole** Hole drilled in the skull.

# C

**Café-au-lait patches** Brown skin patches in neurofibromatosis.

**Canalization** Act of directing into channels.

**Capgras syndrome** Delusion of doubles.

**Capsule** Fibrous barrier around a tumour or abscess.

**Carbon dioxide therapy** Inhalation of a mixture of 30 per cent $CO_2$ and 70 per cent $O_2$ to the point of unconsciousness. Useful in anxiety state and hysterical reactions.

**Caste** Group separated from others by social, racial or religious barriers.

**Castastrophic reaction** Feeling of inadequacy and anxiety to cope with the problem.

**Castration complex** Infantile fear of losing the genital organs.

**Catalepsy** *See* flexibilities cerea.

**Catatonia** State of profound mental automatism or absence of voluntary activity, together with a tendency to immobility and negativism.

**Catatonic stupor** State of intense psychic inhibition during which regression may occur to an infantile or more primitive level, manifest by complete suppression of speech, movement and action.

**Catharsis**   Release of repressed emotion. Approximately synonymous with abreaction.

**Cauda equina**   Nerve fibres lying below the spinal cord.

**Cephalgia**   Headache.

**Cephalic index**   Ratio of breadth to length of the head multiplied by 100.

**Cerebral**   Concerning the brain.

**Cerebral cortex**   Outer surface or layer of the brain composed of grey matter which is infolded to increase its area.

**Cerebral dominance**   One or other lateral half of the cerebral cortex is normally the dominant one.

**Cerebral palsy**   Weakness of various muscle groups due to damage to the brain. Many forms exist. Patients are often referred to as spastics.

**Certification**   Individual legally hospitalized and detained for psychiatric treatment. (*Syn*. compulsory detention.)

**Cervical spondylosis**   Disorder resulting from chronic cervical disc degeneration. Symptoms depend on whether the protrusion is lateral or dorsomedial. Highest incidence from 60 to 70 years of age.

**Chain reaction**   Group associations consisting of linked individual contributions occurring within the group, which is equivalent to 'free association' of psychoanalysis.

**Character**   Sum total of individual's personality.

**Charcot's joints**   Painless disorganized joints in tabes.

**Chasmus hystericus**   Persistent yawning, usually on a hysterical basis.

**Chiasma**   The X-like crossing of the two optic nerves.

**Chorea**   Motor disorder characterized by jerky spasmodic movements. There are two common types: Sydenham's, of rheumatic origin, and Huntington's, hereditary.

**Choreic**   Involuntary movements of an irregular, jerky type, occurring in certain organic brain disorders.

**Choreo-athetotic**   Combination of choreic jerks with the recurring, slow writhing movements of athetosis, resulting from organic brain disease.

**Choroid plexus**   Tufts of vascular tissue in the ventricles of the brain forming the CSF.

**Chromosomes**   Very small bodies contained in the nuclei of cells. The normal human complement is 23 pairs of chromosomes which carry the genetic material·responsible for controlling the development of cells and thus of the whole organism.

**Chronic**   Applied to illness of long duration.

**Chvostek's sign**   Tap over the facial nerve in front of the ear induces a spasm in latent tetany.

**Circle of Willis**   Arterial circle at the base of the brain.

**Circumstantiality**   Long-winded speech.

**Clang associations**   Formed on the basis of rhyme or sound.

**Classical conditioning**   Process of a response to a new stimulus, originally developed by Ivan Petrovich Pavlov.

**Clavus hystericus**   Sensation of a nail being hammered through the skull. Occurs in hysteria.

**Climacteric**   Menopause in women.

**Clitoris**   Female organ, analogue of the penis.

**Clonus**   Rapid intermittent involuntary contraction and relaxation.

**Clouding of consciousness**   Sensorium is not clear.

**Clownism**  Grotesque attitude by psychiatric patients, e.g. buffoonery syndrome in schizophrenia.

**CNS**  Central nervous system.

**Co-conscious**  According to Morton Prince it includes the conscious states that one is not aware of because it is not in the focus of attention but in the fringe of the content of consciousness (Cocs).

**Cognition**  Knowing; thought processes.

**Coitus**  Sexual intercourse per vaginum between male and female.

**Coitus more ferarum**  'Sexual intercourse in the manner of beasts'; buggery.

**Coitus oralis**  Fellatio.

**Collective unconscious**  According to Jung, that part of the unconscious mind inherited from the experiences of the human ràce. (*Syn.* racial unconscious; Cucs.)

**Coma**  Deep loss of consciousness.

**Combat fatigue**  Extreme fatigue resulting from the stress of battle conditions.

**Common group tension**  Effect of pressure underlying shared unconscious fantasies of the members in a group which influences the course of the group associations.

**Communication**  Every event occurring within the group that can be noticed, whether verbal or non-verbal, conscious or unconscious.

**Compensation**  Disguising an undesirable trait by a desirable one, usually of a contrasting nature.

**Complex**  Repressed ideas possessing unconscious activities.

**Compulsion**  Continuous preoccupation with impulse or movement to the exclusion of most other interests, associated with a feeling of compulsion against internal resistance and to the distress of the patient. Occurs normally in play of children, superstitions of adults, rituals of primitive people and contrast ideas, e.g. impulse to swear in the Church; and abnormally as a secondary symptom in chronic schizophrenia, epileptic equivalent, chronic encephalitis lethargica and presenile and senile states. (*Syn.* obsessive-compulsive state.)

**Compulsory detention**   *See* certification.

**Conation**   Doing; acting; behaviour.

**Conditioning**   Ways in which human beings and animals can be systemically taught to respond in a particular manner to stimuli of one sort or another. In Pavlov's classical experiment a dog was conditioned to salivate by giving food at the same time as a bell was rung; then when the bell only was rung it still salivated – a conditioned response.

**Confabulation**   Fabrications to fill memory gaps.

**Conflict**   Conflict between the demands of reality and those of unconscious drives and feelings. This can lead to anxiety and other forms of emotional disorders, the cause not being consciously understood by the subject.

**Confusion**   State of disordered orientation; clouding of consciousness.

**Congenital**   Abnormal conditions present at birth; inborn.

**Conjugate ocular spasm**   *See* oculo-gyric crisis.

**Conscious**   Aware; waking state of the mind; division of the psyche. (Cs.)

**Constitution**   Sum of the physical and mental qualities.

**Conversion**   Transformation of repressed conflict or affect into a physical manifestation, as in hysteria.

**Convolution**   *See* Gyrus.

**Convulsions**   Major epileptic fits.

**Co-ordination**   Smooth and efficient movement.

**Coprolalia**   Utterance of obscene words or phrases.

**Corneal reflex**   Blinking of both the eyelids when the cornea, and not the conjunctiva, is touched with a wisp of cotton-wool brought from the side of the face. Indicates the level of unconsciousness.

**Cortex**   Surface layer of the cerebral and cerebellar hemispheres.

**Co-therapy**   Two people share the responsibility of group leadership, with the advantages of mutual support and the possibilities for discussion of the group experience.

**Counter-transference**   Emotional responses of the therapist to his patient or group, or their transferences to him. It may be a valid and appropriate response, but alternatively it may be the expression of the therapist's own unresolved conflicts.

**Court of protection**   Judicial body whose function is to manage and administer the property and affairs of mentally disordered who cannot do themselves.

**Couvade syndrome**   Psychogenic disorder which affects husbands during their wives' pregnancies or parturition like morning sickness or labour pains.

**Cranial nerves**   Twelve pairs arising from the brain and brain stem.

**Cremasteric reflex**   Contraction of the cremaster on stroking the inner side of the thigh. (L 1.)

**Creutzfeldt–Jakob's disease**   *See* Jakob–Creutzfeldt's disease.

**Cri du chat syndrome**   Mew like a cat. Occurs in severe subnormality with chromosomal abnormality.

**Crime**   Legal wrong, the remedy for which is the punishment of the offender by the State. Legal wrongs may be civil or criminal.

**Criminal responsibility**  Defence on the grounds of insanity has to clearly prove under the McNaughton's Rules that, at the time of committing the act, the accused was labouring under some mental disorder, such that he did not know the nature of the act, or if he did know, he did not know that what he was doing was wrong.

**Crisis intervention**  Transitional period in life or turning point in a disease. There are two categories of crises: 1 developmental; and 2 accidental. The phases of crisis are: 1 impact; 2 recoil; and 3 adjustment. The crisis is resolved with the help of the Services and the caring society.

**CSF**  Cerebrospinal fluid, bathing brain and spinal cord.

**Cunnilingus**  Apposition of the mouth to the female genitals.

**Cybernetics**  Term originally applied in engineering. Introduced by Robert Wiener during the 1940s, referring to the study of automatic message control in the nervous system. Communication and information theory use many cybernetic concepts such as feedback.

**Cyclothymia**  Recurrent mood swings of abnormal degree (depression, elation or both), and not related to external circumstances. Individuals with a tendency to spontaneous mood swings are described as having a 'cyclothymic' personality.

# D

**Da Costa's syndrome**  Derangement of the circulatory system in the absence of objective signs of disease and associated with a desire to escape from the environment. (Syn., effort syndrome; disordered action of the heart.)

**De Clérambault's syndrome**  Woman who has a delusional belief that a man, usually of higher social status and much older in age, is deeply in love with her. Also known as *psychose passionnelle* and erotomania.

**Deep reflexes**   Postural response depending on the stimulation of muscle spindle when a skeletal muscle is stretched, e.g. ankle, biceps, knee, supinator and triceps reflexes.

**Defence**   Process of dealing with feelings, such as anxiety or guilt, by means of mental mechanisms.

**Defence mechanism**   Means by which the organism protects itself against impulses and affects.

**Degeneration**   Death of tissue, often of unknown cause.

**Déjà-vu**   Sense of familiarity.

**Delirium**   State of clouded consciousness with confusion and disorientation, often due to an acute febrile illness or to drugs acting on the brain. Can also occur in various forms of acute brain disease.

**Delusion**   False belief which, in the face of contrary evidence, is held with conviction and is unmodifiable by appeals to reason or logic that would be acceptable to other persons of the same religious or cultural background. Delusions may be classified by: 1 mode of origin; 2 content; and 3 degree of systematization.

**Dementia**   Irreversible impairment of intellectual ability, memory and personality, due to permanent damage or disease of the brain. The term should not be applied to intellectual impairment resulting from temporary or potentially recoverable conditions, as in such cases the patient may afterwards regain his original level of intellectual ability.

**Dementia paralytica**   *See* G.P.I.

**Demyelination**   Loss of the myelin sheath.

**Denial**   Defence mechanism by which a painful experience is rejected.

**Depersonalization**   State in which the individual experiences a change in himself as a loss of his own identity or reality.

## DEPRESSION

**Depression** 1 State of morbid sadness; 2 lowering of mood; and 3 'depression' with psychomotor retardation.

**Derealization** Feeling that the environment is unreal, usually occurs with depersonalization.

**Dereistic thinking** Autistic thinking.

**Dermographia** Elevation on the skin caused by writing on it. A hysterical manifestation.

**Deterioration** Impairment of emotional and higher mental aspects of personality.

**Developmental** Used in a special sense to describe certain disorders which are considered to be primarily anomalies of the development of normal function, e.g. speech.

**Diabetes insipidus** Passage of a large amount of sugar-free urine.

**Diagnosis** Deduction of the nature of neurological or psychiatric disorder from the history, the signs and symptoms and the investigations of the patient.

**Dialogue** Conversation between two or more persons. The ancients taught that after mathematics we need to learn dialogue or discourse – 'the supreme science' as Plato called it. Monologue refers to soliloquy, and dualogue to a dialogue between two people.

**Didactic** Literally, intended to teach; in groups implying a formalized leader-centred teaching situation as distinct from the group-association technique which relies on the group learning from its own experience.

**Diminished responsibility** Where a person kills or is a party to the killing of another, he shall not be convicted if he was suffering from such abnormality of mind (whether arising from a condition of arrested or retarded development of the mind or any inherent causes or induced by disease or injury) as substantially impaired his mental responsibility for his acts and omission in doing or being a party to the killing.

**Diplopia**   Double vision, or the perception of two images for one external object, generally due to a lack of co-ordination between the movements of two eyes.

**Dipsomania**   Recurrent urge to consume alcohol until intoxicated. Occurs in psychopaths rather than alcohol addicts.

**Discriminative sense**   Ability to detect difference in size, shape, texture and number of stimuli.

**Disorientation**   Confusion as to time, place and person.

**Displacement**   Transference of affect from one idea to another to which it does not belong, particularly in a dream.

**Disseminated sclerosis**   Characterized by scattered foci of demyelination of axons and subsequent gliosis throughout the nervous system with remissions and relapses; gradually developing Charcot's classical triad of intention tremors, nystagmus and scanning speech; and ending in paraplegia. (*Syn.*, multiple sclerosis.)

**Dissociated sensory loss**   Loss of pain sense with light touch preserved.

**Dissociation**   Mental mechanism whereby certain aspects or activities of the personality escape from control of the individual. Occurs in conversation hysteria.

**Distractibility**   Tendency for the attention to be easily drawn away from its focus by external diverting stimuli.

**Divorce**   There is only one ground for divorce – irretrievable breakdown of the marriage -- and there are five proofs of such breakdown: 1 one party has committed adultery and the other finds it intolerable to continue the marriage; 2 the behaviour of one partner is so bad that the other cannot reasonably be expected to continue cohabitation; 3 desertion for two years; 4 separate living for two years and a mutual consent for a decree; and 5 separate living for five years. There is no mention of insanity.

**Dominant**  Term used in genetics for a trait which is manifested when the factor or gene concerned is carried on only one of a pair of chromosomes. By comparison a recessive trait is only manifested when the trait is carried on both members of a pair of chromosomes.

**Dominant hemisphere**  Cerebral hemisphere controlling speech.

**Dorsiflexion**  Bending backwards, usually wrist or ankle.

**Double bind**  Term referring to incompatible contradictory emotional demands, made typically by the mother on the child and from which there is no escape, other than withdrawal into a psychotic state, e.g. a childhood experience which might later lead to the development of schizophrenia.

**Down's syndrome**  Caused by an extra chromosome in pair 21 (trisomy 21) making a total of 47 chromosomes. There are two types, regular and translocation. (*Syn.* mongolism.)

**Dream work**  Mechanisms operating to disguise the dream's latent content. They are: 1 dramatization; 2 condensation; 3 displacement; and 4 secondary elaboration.

**Drive**  General term for impulses or motivating forces that prompt an animal towards a goal.

**Drivel**  Grammatically well formed sentences, but the contents are nonsensical. Occurs in schizophrenia and mental subnormality.

**Drop attacks**  Sudden falls with loss of consciousness; akinetic epilepsy.

**Drug dependence**  'State of periodic or chronic intoxication, detrimental to the individual and to society, produced by the repeated consumption of a drug'. (WHO, 1964; *Cf.* addiction; habituation.)

**Dura mater**  Outer-most layer of meninges.

**Durham test**  U.S. Court of Appeals in 1954 gave the ruling that the accused is not criminally responsible if his unlawful act was the product of mental disease or mental defect.

**Dynamic**   Term describing an approach both to psychology and sociology, essentially involving change and interaction in contrast to static descriptive approaches.

**Dysarthria**   Impairment of speech or articulation due to disease of the muscles of speech.

**Dyslalia**   Form of dysarthria in which infantile modes of articulation persist to an abnormally late age.

**Dyslexia**   Inability to read at a level appropriate to the individual's age and intelligence.

**Dysmetria**   Inability to arrest a muscular movement at a desired point; past-pointing.

**Dysmnesia**   Impaired or disordered memory. Occurs in organic brain disorder.

**Dyspareunia**   Difficult or painful intercourse in the female.

**Dysphasia**   Partial loss of speech.

**Dyssynergia**   Unison movements, involving more than one joint, are broken up into their component parts. They resemble the jerky movements of a puppet.

**Dysthymia**   Depression associated with hypochondriacal symptoms.

**Dystonic reactions**   Abnormal muscular tension. Occurs in akathisia and Parkinsonism as a complication of drug therapy.

**Dystrophy**   Degeneration with loss of function.

# E

**Echo de la pensée**   Echoing of the thoughts.

**Echolalia**   Repetition of words or phrases spoken to the individual.

**Echopraxia**  Repetition of the acts of another person.

**Ecstasy**  Rapturous joy.

**ECT**  Electroconvulsive therapy was introduced in 1938 by Ugo Cerletti for the treatment of psychiatric disorders like endogenous depression, mania, toxic confusional states and certain forms of schizophrenia. The different types of ECT are: 1 straight; 2 bilateral; and 3 unilateral. For some obscure reason this treatment has recently received adverse publicity. (*Syn.* electroplexy.)

**Effector**  Nerve ending in a muscle or gland.

**Ego**  Part of the mind that is experienced by the individual as his 'self' and which, under the guidance of the 'super-ego' is concerned with satisfying the unconscious primitive demands of the 'id' in such a way that their experience is acceptable in a socially approved form. Characteristics of ego are: it is conscious, logical, moral and controlled by super-ego; sleeps but maintains dream censorship.

**Ego ideal**  Standards that the individual tries to achieve.

**Eidetic imagery**  Brilliant mental pictures that can be recalled in the mind. Common in children but rare in adults.

**Elation**  Happy mood; feeling of buoyancy.

**Electra complex**  Female equivalent of the Oedipus complex. The girl wishes to displace her mother and possess her father.

**Electrocardiograph**  Record of the electrical impulses arising from the heart muscles (ECG; EKG).

**Electrocorticography**  Recording electrical activity direct from the cortex (ECoG).

**Electroencephalograph**  Record of the variations in electrical potential between different parts of the brain. Normally a number of channels are recorded simultaneously using electrodes placed at different points on the skull (EEG).

**Electromyography**  Recording the electrical activity of muscle (EMG).

**Electroplexy**  Electroconvulsive therapy (ECT).

**Emotion**  Stirred up state of mind and/or body. (*Cf.* affect, feeling, mood, sentiment, passion.)

**Empathy**  When an observer is able to enter into the thoughts and feelings of the patient and establish a good contact.

**Encephalitis**  Inflammation of the brain. (*Pl.* encephalitudes.)

**Encephalopathy**  Disorder of brain function.

**Encopresis**  Incontinence of faeces.

**Endocrine**  Applied to the system of ductless glands. The internal secretions or hormones which they produce are of great importance in controlling development and bodily functions.

**Endogenous**  This means originating from within; and exogenous, originating from without. Used in psychiatry to distinguish between the depressive illnesses, but most depressions show evidence of both endogenous and exogenous factors.

**Endogenous depression**  Affective disorder due to a hereditary predisposition. Depression arising from within the person.

**Enuresis**  Incontinence of urine.

**Environment**  Sum total of the surroundings.

**Epilepsy**  Episodic abnormality of the brain function with loss of consciousness, which may or may not be associated with tonic spasm and clonic contractions of the muscles. Also described as 'paroxysmal cerebral dysrhythmia' (Gibbs, Gibbs and Lennox, 1937). Epilepsy is a symptom as well as a disease; and depends upon the individual's convulsive threshold. (*Syn.* grand mal.)

**Epiloia**  Condition characterized by mental deficiency, skin rash, epilepsy and tumours in the brain and body. (*Syn.* tuberose sclerosis.)

**Episode**  Transistory phase in a disorder.

**Euphoria**  Feelings of well-being; more than elation.

**Exaltation**  Intense elation.

**Exhibitionist**  Person who obtains sexual pleasure by exposing his genital organs to other people.

**Existential**  Term now employed in psychiatry giving priority to total subjective experience or 'being', as distinct from underlying forces or casual explanations.

**Exogenous**  *See* Endogenous.

**Experimental neurosis**  Neurosis produced in animals by introducing conflicting responses to stimuli.

**Extensor plantar response**  Big toe goes up on scratching the sole.

**Extinction**  Abolition of learned response, normally achieved by withholding reinforcement.

**Extracranial**  Outside the skull.

**Extradural**  Between the dura and the skull.

**Extrapyramidal**  Motor fibres arising from cells other than the pyramidal cells (often basal ganglia).

**Extrasensory perception**  Controversial category of experience consisting of perception not mediated by sense-organ stimulation, for example, clairvoyance and telepathy (ESP).

**Extrinsic**  Outside and separate from nervous tissue.

**Eysenck personality inventory**  Questionnaire giving scores for extraversion and neuroticism (EPI).

# F

**Fabrication**  Act of replacing memory loss by phantasy. (*Syn.* confabulation.)

**Facial nerve**  Seventh, mixed nerve: motor part supplies the muscles of facial expression and the sensory carries the sense of taste from the front of the tongue.

**Fallacy**  Error in reasoning.

**False statements**  Wilfully making false statements with an intent to deceive.

**Fantasy**  Production of mental images to provide gratification or satisfaction often not obtainable in reality.

**Faradic shock**  Electric shock used in aversion therapy.

**Fasciculation**  Involuntary twitching of isolated bundles of muscle fibres.

**Father surrogate**  Father substitute. (*Cf.* mother surrogate.)

**Feeblemindedness**  Term for mental subnormality. (*Syn.* moron.)

**Feedback**  Term borrowed from cybernetic theory and now used in psychosocial situations such as therapeutic groups.

**Feeling**  Emotion, mood, affect.

**Fellatio**  Application of mouth to the penis.

**Fetishism**  Person sexually aroused by objects not regarded as sexually stimulating.

**Fibrillation**  Contractions of individual muscle fibres. Cannot be detected clinically but may be recorded by the electro-myograph.

**Figure-ground**  Perceptions are patterned into two aspects: 1 the figure, which stands out; and 2 matrix, which forms the ground. (*Syn.* shifting perception.)

2

**Fissure**   Groove on the surface of the brain. (*Syn.* sulcus; *Pl.* sulci.)

**Fitness to plead**   Criteria of fitness to plead are: 1 the prisoner should be able to instruct his Counsel; 2 he should appreciate the significance of pleading 'Guilty' or 'Not Guilty'; 3 he should be able to challenge a juror; 4 he should be able to examine witnesses; and 5 he should be able to understand and follow the evidence placed before the Court, and Court procedure.

**Fits**   Convulsions; seizures.

**Fixation**   1 Persistent behaviour which is no longer useful; and 2 the strengthening of learned habit.

**Flaccid**   Limp; floppy; loss of tone.

**Flagellation**   Erotic pleasure derived from whipping. A female flagellator is called fouetteuse.

**Flattening of affect**   Emotional shallowness which is a feature of schizophrenia.

**Flexibilitas cerea**   Condition in which the body and the limbs remain in the position in which they have been placed. Occurs in catatonic schizophrenia. (*Syn.* catalepsy; wax-like rigidity; Egyptian-mummy attitude.)

**Flexor plantar response**   Normal downward movement of the big toe on scratching the foot.

**Flexor spasm**   Painful contractions of muscles in spastic limbs.

**Flight of ideas**   Succession of thoughts with no rational connection. Clang associations also occur. Typical of hypomania and mania.

**Flooding**   Patient is exposed to the situation which makes him anxious until he is able to feel anxious no longer. (*Syn.* implosion therapy.)

**Focal**   Arising from, or limited to, one part.

**Focal epilepsy**  Fit arising from one point in the brain. (*Syn.* Jacksonian epilepsy.)

**Folie à deux**  Sharing of delusions by two closely associated individuals, such as husband and wife, one of whom suffers from a paranoid illness and eventually succeeds in inducing similar delusions in the other. (Folie à trois, i.e. with three people.)

**Folie circulaire**  'Cyclic insanity' now known as manic-depressive psychosis.

**Folie du doute**  Insanity of doubt. Occurs in doubting mania of obsessive–compulsive state.

**Folie du toucher**  Compulsive behaviour to touch certain objects.

**Folie raisonnante**  'Reasoning insanity'. Occurs in hypomania.

**Foramen**  Opening; aperture.

**Forensic**  Pertaining to law of courts and legal procedures.

**Forgery**  Making of a false document in order that it may be used as genuine with intent to deceive or defraud the public.

**Formes frustes**  Atypical symptoms of a disease.

**Formication**  Feeling as if insects were crawling all over the body. Occurs in delirium tremens; and 'cocaine bugs'. (*Cf.* signe de Magnan.)

**Fortication spectra**  Zig-zag patterns seen in migraine.

**Fossa**  Compartment of the skull holding a part of the brain.

**Fragmentation**  Molecular splitting of the psyche. Characteristic of schizophrenia.

**Free-association**  Patient during psychoanalysis is encouraged to express freely whatever thoughts or ideas that come into his mind. Thus, the unconscious material may be recalled.

**Free-floating anxiety** Unresolved fear associated with any situation.

**Freudian** Descriptive term for the school of psychoanalysis by Sigmund Freud (1856–1939). It is today widely applied to other fields of psychiatry, including group psychotherapy.

**Frigidity** Inability of the woman to achieve an orgasm through coitus. Similar condition in the male is termed impotence.

**Fröhlich syndrome** Adiposogenital is characterized by obesity and underdevelopment of the gonads. Lesion is in the hypothalamus.

**Frontal lobe syndrome** Facetious, irresponsible and anti-social behaviour.

**Frustration** Thwarting of a drive leading to aggression, regression, fixation and finally resignation.

**Fugue** State of alteration of consciousness combined with an impulse to wander. Occurs in hysteria, depression, epilepsy, schizophrenia, organic cerebral disease and psychopathy.

**Function** Activity of an object which fulfils some purpose.

**Functional psychosis** Grave mental disorder without organic basis.

# G

**Gag reflex** Touching the posterior wall of the pharynx is followed by constriction and elevation of the pharynx.

**Galvanic skin response** Changes in the electric resistance of the skin as detected by galvanometer. (*Syn.* psychogalvanic response.)

**Gamete** Sex cell which when united with another sex cell forms a zygote.

**Ganglia** Collection of nerve cells.

**Ganser syndrome** State of approximate answers similar to hysterical pseudodementia.

**GBH** Grievous bodily harm.

**Gene** Unit of a chromosome responsible for reproducing the characteristics of the cell on division.

**Generalization** 1 Response to the new stimulus similar to the training stimulus; 2 broad principle in science.

**Generalized fits** Convulsions affecting all parts of the body.

**Gerstmann's syndrome** Damage to the dominant angular gyrus of the parietal lobe resulting in agraphia, acalculia, finger agnosia and right–left disorientation.

**Gessell's development scales** Mental ability test for assessment of mental growth in children.

**Gestalt** Integrated whole which is greater than the sum of its parts. (*Cf.* pattern, configuration; *Pl.* Gestalten.)

**Gestalt psychology** School of psychology which favours the perception of a Gestalt or a whole rather than its parts. The chief exponents of Gestalt school were Max Wertheimer, Wolfgang Kohler and Kurt Kaffka.

**Gibson spiral maze test** Assesses psychomotor accuracy and speed.

**Gilles de la Tourette syndrome** Involuntary movements with compulsive shouting, usually of obscene nature. (*Syn.* lata.)

**Girdle pains** Constricting pains around the trunk.

**Gjessing's syndrome** Mental changes associated with variations in nitrogen retention in periodic catatonic schizophrenia.

**Glabellar reflex** Tap over the root of the nose with a finger results in the nasopalpebral response of bilateral blinking of the eyelids. This is a confirmatory sign of extrapyramidal disease.

**Glia**  Supporting cells and fibres of the nervous system.

**Glioblastoma**  Malignant glioma.

**Glioma**  Tumour growing from the supporting cells.

**Gliosis**  Overgrowth of glial fibres.

**Globus hystericus**  Lump in the throat; sensation of a lump arising from the stomach to the throat.

**Glossopharyngeal nerve**  Ninth, mixed nerve supplies the muscles of the pharynx and carries the sensation of taste from the posterior third of the tongue.

**Glove and stocking anaesthesia**  Impaired sensation over the periphery of all four limbs.

**Goldstein–Scheerer test**  Assesses abstract ability. Diagnostic of brain damage.

**GPI**  General paralysis of the insane. This is caused by syphilis of the nervous system. (*Syn.* dementia paralytica.)

**Grafted schizophrenia**  Schizophrenic syndrome grafted upon intellectual deficiency. (*Syn.* Propf schizophrenia.)

**Gramophone symptom**  Pathognomonic of Pick's disease. The patient repeats with correct expression and diction an elaborate anecdote without stop; and then after a short interval he repeats the anecdote as something quite new.

**Grand mal**  Generalized convulsion with loss of consciousness. (*Syn.* epilepsy.)

**Grasp reflex**  Object placed in patient's hand elicits a tonic contraction of the flexor muscles which is increased on an attempt to withdraw it. Occurs in lesions of the prefrontal lobes.

**Grey matter**  Nervous tissue containing nerve cells.

**Grid technique**  Application and recording of the individual's constructs in the interview situation.

**Grief**  Profound sadness.

**Group**  Number of individuals connected for some purpose or circumstance.

**Group content**  Consists of the ideas, feelings and attitudes which emerge through the group processes.

**Group matrix**  Total communication network within the group.

**Group process**  Method by which group resolves problems and meet objectives.

**Group psychotherapy**  Group meeting of patients with the therapist. The object is to achieve mental catharsis.

**Group structure**  Physical arrangement of the group. A small group consists of six or seven members, and along with the conductor are seated in a circle.

**Growth hormone**  Substance produced by the pituitary gland. Insufficient production of the hormone leads to retarded growth; and excessive, to increased growth, sometimes to abnormally great stature.

**Guilty mind**  Mens rea; malice aforethought.

**Gyrus**  Fold on the surface of the cerebral cortex. (*Syn.* convolution; *Pl.* gyri.)

# H

**Habit**  Acquired response learned by repetition of certain stimuli.

**Habituation**  Psychological dependence upon drugs like tobacco and cannabis. (*Cf.* addiction; drug dependence.)

**Hallucination**  False perception without external stimulation. Any of the senses may be involved, so that a hallucination can mean seeing, hearing, smelling, tasting or feeling something that is not actually present, and are named accordingly, e.g. visual, auditory, olfactory, gustatory and tactile hallucinations. As there is a shift from the unconscious to the conscious, hallucinations are found in normal individuals between the sleeping and waking state, but they are characteristic of some of the psychiatric disorders.

**Hamilton rating scales**  These are for depression and anxiety. 1 For depression it consists of the following 17 items: depressed mood, guilt, suicidal ideas, initial insomnia, middle insomnia, delayed insomnia, work and interests, retardation, agitation, psychic anxiety, somatic anxiety, gastro-intestinal somatic symptoms, general somatic symptoms, genital symptoms, hypochondriasis, loss of insight and loss of weight. 2 For anxiety it includes 12 features: anxious mood, tension, fears, insomnia, intellect, depressed mood, general somatic, cardiovascular, respiratory, gastrointestinal, genito-urinary, autonomic and behaviour.

**Haptic**  Cutaneous sensations that may be hallucinatory.

**Hebephrenia**  Chronic form of schizophrenia.

**Hedonism**  Theory that man seeks pleasure and avoids pain; and pleasure or happiness is the highest good.

**Hemianopia**  Loss of half of the visual field.

**Hemiballism**  Violent limb movements of wide amplitude to the other side of the body.

**Hemiplegia**  Paralysis of one half of the body.

**Heredity**  Individual characteristics passed on genetically by parents to their offspring.

**Heredo-familial**  Passed from generation to generation and to several members of one family.

**Herpes zoster**  Viral infection of posterior root ganglia resulting in pain and rash over the corresponding cutaneous distribution of the affected nerve root.

**Heterosexual**  Sexual attraction towards persons of the opposite sex.

**Heterozygous twins**   Twins that are dissimilar.

**Hiatus**   Large gap.

**Hierarchial**   Descriptive of an organization involving levels of ascending authority and power; it is a term often used in relation to hospital structures and systems of communications.

**Hoffmann's sign**   Flicking the nail of the patient's middle finger results in a prompt adduction of the thumb and flexion of the index finger. Caused by injury to the pyramidal tract.

**Holmes–Adie's syndrome**   Response of the pupil to accommodation and light is extremely slow. $(A - R -)$. The pupils are usually unequal; and deep reflexes are absent. Aetiology is unknown.

**Homicide**   Killing of a human being by another human being. A person of sound mind and discretion unlawfully kills any human creature in being and under the Queen's peace with malice aforethought.

**Homonymous**   Same on both sides.

**Homosexual**   Sexual attraction towards persons of the same sex.

**Hormic psychology**   McDougall's psychology of instincts.

**Hormone**   Substance produced by an endocrine gland.

**Horner's syndrome**   Caused by paralysis of the cervical sympathetic. Signs and symptoms are: 1 miosis; 2 enophthalmos; 3 pseudoptosis; and 4 vasodilation and anhidrosis on the same side of the face and neck.

**Hostile aggression**   One whose primary aim is to inflict injury.

**Housebound syndrome**   Agoraphobia.

**Huntington's chorea**   Hereditary disease of the nervous system characterized by jerky movements.

**Hyperacusis** Hyperaesthesia of the auditory nerve. Slight sounds are heard with painful intensity. Occurs in lesion of the facial nerve and hysteria.

**Hyperkinesis** Excessive motor activity, often with little apparent purpose.

**Hyperphagia** Pathological overeating.

**Hypertonia** Increased tone of the muscles of the limb; spasticity. The various forms of hypertonia are: 1 clasp-knife rigidity: initial resistance which suddenly gives way; 2 cog-wheel rigidity: intermittently normal and increased tone; and 3 lead-pipe or plastic rigidity: increased resistance throughout the movement.

**Hypertrophy** Enlargement.

**Hyperventilation** Excessively deep and fast breathing.

**Hypnagogic** Inducing sleep; hypnotic.

**Hypnoanalysis** Use of hypnosis for the analysis of the mind.

**Hypnopompic** Sleep-dispelling; waking up.

**Hypnosis** Temporary condition of altered attention in the subject which may be induced by another person and in which a variety of phenomena may appear spontaneously or in response to verbal or other stimuli. These phenomena include alterations in consciousness and memory, increased susceptibility to suggestion, and the production in the subject of responses and ideas unfamiliar to him in his mind. Further, phenomena such as anaesthesia, paralysis, muscle rigidity and vasomotor changes can be produced and removed in hypnotic state.

**Hypnotic** Drug producing sleep.

**Hypochondriasis** 1 False belief in the actual presence of physical disease; and 2 mental preoccupation with an unreal (or, if real, exaggerated) or supposed physical disorder.

**Hypoglossal nerve**   Twelfth, motor nerve which supplies the muscles of the tongue.

**Hypoglycaemia**   Abnormally low blood sugar.

**Hypomania**   Milder form of mania.

**Hypopituitarism**   Lack of pituitary function.

**Hysteria**   Purposive functional disability in which two different types of reaction may occur: 1 conversion reaction with disturbances of physical functions, e.g. functional paralysis; and (2) dissociative reaction with disturbances of consciousness, memory and behaviour, e.g. amnesia, fugue and Ganser syndrome.

# I

**Iatrogenic**   Applied signs and symptoms or illness unintentionally produced either directly as a result of treatment given or indirectly through remarks overheard by the patient regarding investigations.

**Id**   Psychoanalytic concept of the unconscious mind containing the main driving force of the individual in the form of primitive impulses, the satisfaction of which is regulated by the ego in such a way as to avoid conflict with the dictates of super-ego. The characteristic of Id are: it is unconscious, amoral, illogical and seat of pleasure–pain principle; reservoir of libido and phylogenetic deposits.

**Ideas of reference**   Person may have quite unfounded ideas that others are referring to him in their speech, writings and gestures.

**Identification**   Acquisition of the views and attitudes of another person as a result of a close, usually loving or admiring, relationship with that person; an emotional tie.

**Idiopathic**   Pathological condition in which no cause can be discovered. Condition with known aetiology is described as symptomatic. Thus epilepsy is termed idiopathic in the absence of any recognizable cause, and symptomatic when due to some cerebral lesion.

**Idiot**   Grade of mental deficiency; severe subnormality with IQ below 25.

**Illusion**   False perception with external stimulation. Illusion should be distinguished from hallucination and like it may involve any of the senses. Illusion is more common at night and generally occurs in a state of altered consciousness.

**Imagery**   Projections of perceptions in the mind so that mental pictures can be experienced.

**Imagination**   Conscious formation of new ideas or concepts based on past experience.

**Imbecile**   Grade of mental deficiency; severe subnormality with a mental age of 3 to 7 years and IQ between 26 and 50.

**Implosion therapy**   Behaviour therapy in which a phobia is treated by repeatedly presenting anxiety-arousing stimuli until the anxiety is extinguished. (*Syn.* flooding.)

**Impotence**   Partial or total inability of the male to achieve and maintain an erection during sexual intercourse.

**Impulses**   Electrical waves travelling along nerves.

**Inborn**   Part of an individual's make-up.

**Incoherence**   Absence of an orderly flow of ideas.

**Incongruity of affect**   Disharmony between the patient's affective state and accompanying thought content which may be a feature in some cases of schizophrenia.

**Individual psychology**   School of psychology developed by Alfred Adler.

**Industrial therapy**   Variety of measures designed to fit the long-stay patients in a psychiatric hospital.

**Inhibition**   Stopping of an ongoing process; mental blockage; the prevention of libidinal impulses from reaching consciousness.

**Innate**   Inborn or hereditary in contrast to acquired.

**Intelligence**   General all round ability to perform mental tasks.

**Intelligence quotient**   Index of a person's relative level of brightness as compared with others of his age; and expressed by the formula:

$$IQ = \frac{MA}{CA} \times 100$$

where MA is mental age and CA is chronological age.

**Intention tremors**   Rhythmical oscillations of the part of a limb on an attempt to use the affected muscles. It stops at rest and increases in severity as the voluntary movement continues. Occurs in disseminated (multiple) sclerosis.

**Intermittent reinforcement**   Any pattern of reinforcement which is not continuous.

**Interpretation**   Statement offering an understanding of meaning rather than an explanation of cause.

**Intervertebral disc**   Fibro-cartilaginous cushion between the vertebrae.

**Intracranial**   Inside the skull.

**Intracranial hypertension**   High pressure inside the skull (not high blood pressure).

**Intrinsic**   Inside the substance of the nervous system.

**Introjection**   Absorption of environment or the personality of others into one's self, thus producing identification of one's self with other persons or objects. (*Opp.* projection.)

**Introspection**   Observation by an individual of the workings of his own mind and of his feelings and reactions to particular situations, events and people.

**Introvert** Personality characterized by introspection and direction of interest inwards. A shut-in type of personality.

**Involuntary** Not under conscious control.

**Involuntary movements** Muscular activity not under individual's control.

**Involution** Period of life from the age of about 50 years on during which there is a general falling-off in the level of various bodily functions.

**Involutional melancholia** Endogenous depression arising during the period of involution.

**Isolation** Condition of being isolated; habitual avoidance of social contacts; the separation of memories from their emotional components.

# J

**Jacksonian epilepsy** Convulsions localized to one limb or one side of the body, usually without initial loss of consciousness.

**Jakob-Creutzfeldt's disease** Cortico-striato-spinal degeneration. (*Syn.* Creutzfeldt-Jakob's disease.)

**Jaw reflex** Lower jaw with half-open mouth is held between the finger and the thumb. A tap on the thumb elicits the jaw jerk indicating a bilateral upper motor neuron lesion.

**Jungian** Carl Gustav Jung (1875–1961) formed his own school of analytical psychology. Religion, myth, archetypes, collective and racial unconsciousness concepts enter his formulations.

**Jung's free word association test** Projective test where responses to a list of words stimuli are evaluated.

**Jung's types** Personality types like extravert and introvert.

# K

**Kayser-Fleischer ring**  Smoky brownish ring due to deposits of copper at the outer margin of the cornea. Pathognomic of hepatolenticular degeneration (Wilson's disease).

**Kernig's sign**  Attempt to extend the knee while the knee and hip joints are flexed results in a spasm of the hamstring muscles. It is a sign of meningeal irritation.

**Kleinian**  Melanie Klein (1882–1960), a psychoanalyst, who introduced influential theories concerning the psychological development in the first year of life.

**Kleptomania**  Morbid impulse to steal.

**Klinefelter's syndrome**  Chromosomal abnormality with 47 chromosomes. Signs and symptoms include dysgenesis of the seminiferous tubules, gynaecomastia, eunuchoidism and phenotypically to be male. Sex chromatin test is positive. (*Syn.* XXY syndrome.)

**Knee jerk**  Monosynaptic stretch reflex elicited by a tap on the patellar tendon resulting in the contraction of the quadriceps muscle. (L 2, L 3, L 4.)

**Knight's move thinking**  Symbolically from a piece in chess bearing a horse's head which moves one square in a set direction and then one square diagonally from it; derailment; tangency.

**Korsakoff's psychosis**  Chronic alcoholism in which multiple neuritis, memory loss and confabulation occurs. (*Syn.* Korsakov, Korsakow or amnestic syndrome.)

**Kraepelin's disease**  Presenile dementia associated with depressive psychosis and catatonic features. Its independent entity is doubtful.

**Kretschmer's types**  Physical classification of personality into three main types: 1 athletic, strong and muscular; 2 asthenic, thin and delicate; and 3 pyknic, short and stout.

**Kuru** Transmissible spongiform slow virus encephalopathy associated with the ritual cannibalism of human brains in New Guinea. Kuru is analogous to Creutzfeldt-Jakob's disease.

# L

**Lability of affect** Tendency to sudden changes in mood. It occurs in personality disorder and brain damage.

**Labyrinth** Semicircular canals of the inner ear.

**La folie circulaire** 'Recurrent madness'; manic-depressive psychosis.

**Lange curve** Test carried out by adding CSF to colloidal gold solution.

**Lasègue's sign** Limitation of straight leg raising.

**Lawrence–Moon–Biedl syndrome** Recessive gene with subnormality, defective vision, extra fingers or toes, obesity and under-developed sex organs.

**Leader-centred groups** Groups are leader-centred when communication is directed towards the therapist.

**Leadership** Authority in a group to direct its activities.

**Learning** Modification of behaviour as a result of experience.

**Learning theory** Psychological theory which seeks to explain behaviour in terms of learned responses to environment, in contrast to dynamic theory, such as psychoanalysis. It is an extension of the work of Ivan Petrovich Pavlov and provides the theoretical basis for behaviour therapy, in terms of deconditioning and re-learning.

**Leptosome** Kretschmer's asthenic type.

**Lesion** Localized area of tissue damage.

**Libido** Term used for sexual drive and in psychoanalysis, for 'psychic energy'.

**Lightning pains** Needle-like pains in the limbs in tabes.

**Lobe** Major division of the cerebral hemispheres.

**Localize** Determine the exact point affected.

**Logoclonia** Vocal repetition of parts of a word.

**Logorrhoea** Rapid and voluble speech like the non-stop manic chatter.

**Lower motor neurone** Axons of the anterior horn cells of the spinal cord and nuclei of the motor cranial nerves. Signs of a lesion of the lower motor neurone are: 1 paralysis of the muscles; 2 loss of muscle tone (flaccidity); 3 wasting of muscles (atrophy); 4 reflexes: deep, absent; superficial, normal; 5 contractures; 6 fibrillations; 7 reaction of degeneration; and 8 pain.

**Lumbago** Pain in the lower part of the back.

# M

**Macropsia** Illusion where objects appear larger than normal size.

**Maladjusted** Emotionally disturbed children requiring special type of educational provision.

**Malice aforethought** Criminal intention to: 1 kill; 2 inflict grievous bodily harm. It is a distinctive attribute of murder. Malice may be express, implied, transfer or universal.

**Malingerer** One who pretends illness; faking; playing possum.

**Mania** Elation with psychomotor acceleration. (*Opp.* depression.)

**Mania à potu** Transient alcoholic mania in a person susceptible to small amounts of alcohol; pathological intoxication.

## MANIC-DEPRESSIVE

**Manic-depressive** Affective disorder characterized by alternating exaltation and depression.

**Mannerism** Rapidly performed, semi-automatic grimace and/or gesture.

**Masochism** Sexual pleasure obtained by suffering physical pain.

**Masturbation** Self-stimulation of the genitals to induce sexual excitement.

**Maturation** Growth or developmental process.

**Maturity** Completion of development to the accepted norm; puberty.

**McNaughton's rules** Daniel McNaughton (ten different spellings) in 1843 shot and killed Alexander Drummond, private secretary to Sir Robert Peel. He had mistaken Drummond for the latter. McNaughton suffered from delusions of persecution and had finally woven Sir Robert Peel into his delusional system. He was found not guilty, which culminated in a debate in the House of Lords when the now famous McNaughton's Rules were formulated. The Rules stated that in order to establish a defence on grounds of insanity it must be proved: 1 that, at the time of committing the act, the accused was labouring under such a defect of reason from disease of the mind as not to know the nature and quality of the act he was doing or, if he knew what he was doing, he did not know that it was wrong; and 2 if the accused commits an act by reason of delusion, the degree of responsibility is based on the justification which the delusion would provide if it were true. 3 *Note:* everybody is presumed sane until the contrary is proved.

**Medulla** Lowest part of the brain stem.

**Megalomania** Delusions of grandeur.

**Melancholia** Temperament given to depression.

**Memory**  Involves three aspects: 1 registration; 2 retention; and 3 recall.

**Memory for designs test**  Test requiring the reproduction of designs from memory. The performance of brain damaged patient is impaired.

**Menarche**  Beginning of menstrual function which indicates puberty or the start of the reproductive period in the female.

**Ménière's syndrome**  Recurrent paroxyms of vertigo with tinnitus and progressive nerve deafness.

**Meninges**  Three membranes covering the brain and cord and lining the skull and vertebral canal.

**Meningioma**  Benign tumour growing from the arachnoid.

**Meningism**  Sign of irritation of the meninges, not due to infection.

**Meningitis**  Inflammation of the meninges, the membranes covering the brain and spinal cord.

**Meningocoele**  Bulge of the meninges through a breach in the bony coverings.

**Meningo-encephalitis**  Inflammation of both brain and meninges.

**Meningo-mylocoele**  Meningocoele containing spinal cord tissue.

**Menopause**  Cessation of menstrual function which indicates the end of the reproductive period in the female, and is commonly referred to as the change of life.

**Mens rea**  Malice aforethought or guilty mind. A bare intent, however criminal, is not punishable unless followed by a criminal act.

**Mental deficiency**  Old term for mental subnormality.

**Mental hygiene** Investigation and furtherance of measures that tend to preserve and promote mental health.

**Mental mechanisms** Mental devices employed unconsciously to meet the emotional needs and purposes of the personality. Two main groups are described: 1 adjustive, e.g. compensation, conversion, deflection, rationalization and sublimation; 2 refusal, e.g. denial, isolation, regression and withdrawal.

**Micropsia** Illusion where objects appear smaller than normal size.

**Migraine** Severe one-sided headache with painful sensitivity to light (photophobia), visual images resembling the battlements of a castle (castellations) and vomiting. (*Cf.* wonderland syndrome.)

**Mill Hill vocabulary scale** Test of mental achievement by estimating vocabulary.

**Minnesota multiphasic personality inventory** A questionnaire that measures personality traits, and helps in psychiatric diagnosis. (MMPI)

**Mitchell vocabulary test** Ability test of 15 commonly used words with selection of one of four meanings for each word.

**Mixed nerve** One containing motor and sensory fibres.

**Mnemonic systems** Artificial aids to memory.

**Modified new word learning test** Test of brain damage in which the subject is required to learn the meanings of words unfamiliar to him.

**Mongolism** *See* Down's syndrome.

**Monoplegia** Paralysis of one limb.

**Mood** Long drawn-out emotion.

**Moral insanity** Term formerly used to describe psychopathic personalities.

**Morbid**   Abnormal in quality or degree. More prolonged in duration than is normally expected to be, e.g. grief.

**Moron**   Mental subnormality with the highest grade of feeble-mindedness and an IQ between 50 and 70.

**Motivation**   Goal-seeking activity.

**Motive**   Conscious or unconscious reason behind a particular attitude or behaviour; intent – direct or indirect.

**Motor**   Concerned with muscular movement.

**Motor neurone disease**   Degeneration of the motor neurones involving both the corticospinal pathways and also the motor nuclei of the brain-stem and the anterior horn cells of the spinal cord. (*Syn.* amyotrophic lateral sclerosis.)

**Multiple sclerosis**   Disseminated sclerosis.

**Munchausen's syndrome**   Name suggested by Asher in 1951 to patients who gain admission to hospital by feigning acute medical and surgical illnesses. Motive is largely unknown. Hysteria or psychopathy often underlie this condition.

**Murder**   Unlawfully killing a reasonable creature in being and under the Queen's peace with malice aforethought, express or implied, the death following within a year and a day. (*Syn.* homicide.)

**Music therapy**   Different from the routine hospital programme of radio, record-players and cassettes. Manipulation of mood by the use of music is carried out in a matrix of eating, reading, talking and working. The inexhaustible patience of the music therapist leads to the final success. Results of music therapy cannot be specifically assessed because of other therapeutic measures involved. But its practical value cannot be disputed.

**Mutism**   Condition of being without speech.

**Myasthenia**   Weakness of muscle.

**Myasthenia gravis**  Chronic affection of adult life characterized by progressive muscular weakness, beginning usually in the face and throat but unaccompanied by atrophy.

**Myelin**  Substance forming the sheaths of nerves. Loss of the myelin sheaths cause failure of the function of nerves, as in demyelinating diseases.

**Myelitis**  Inflammation of the spinal cord.

**Myelography**  The X-raying of the vertebral canal by introducing opaque fluid into the CSF.

**Myoclonia**  Spasmodic muscular contractions, e.g. myoclonic epilepsy; and petit mal with myoclonia.

**Myopathy**  Degenerative disease of muscle, e.g. muscular dystrophy.

**Myositis**  Inflammation of muscle.

**Myotonia**  Contraction of muscle persisting after the need for it is over.

# N

**Narcissism**  Self-love.

**Narcoanalysis**  Abreaction with a narcotic such as Amytal (amylobarbitone sodium) or Pentothal (sodium thiopentone).

**Narcolepsy**  Sudden desire to sleep.

**Neck rigidity**  Passive flexion of the head results in the spasm of the extensors of the neck. Occurs in the inflammation of the meninges.

**Need**  Requirement for satisfaction.

**Negative practice**  Repetition of behaviour for the purpose of extinguishing it.

**Negative reinforcement** Event whose removal following a response strengthens the tendency of that response to occur. (*Syn.* punishment.)

**Negativism** Doing the opposite.

**Negligence** Noncompliance with a standard of conduct.

**Neologism** Making new meaningless words.

**Neurasthenia** Pathological weakness characterized by physical and mental fatigue.

**Neuritis** Pain in the distribution of a nerve; inflammation of a nerve.

**Neurology** Diseases of the nervous system.

**Neuromuscular junction** Point where a nerve fibre ends in a muscle.

**Neurone** Nerve cell with its processes.

**Neuroses** Disorders of the personality in which instinctive and emotional difficulties are manifested as mental and physical signs and symptoms. (*Syn.* psychoneuroses.)

**Neurosyphilis** Syphilitic involvement of the nervous system.

**Neurotic** Person suffering from neurosis.

**Nightmare** Fright reaction during sleep.

**Nihilism** Delusion of non-existence.

**Nirvana** Death instinct; oblivion to external reality.

**Non compos mentis** 'Not of a sane mind'.

**Nosology** Study of the classification of diseases.

**Nucleus** Collection of nerve cells.

**Nymphomania** Insatiable desire for sex in women.

**Nystagmus** Rhythmical oscillation of the eyes.

# O

**Objective** 1 Something to be aimed at and achieved where possible; and 2 that which can be perceived through the external senses. (*Opp.* subjective.)

**Object relations technique** Projective test using pictures representing people and situations.

**Obscenity** Verbal or written use of words as a means of achieving sexual excitement or inducing it in others, including graffiti, writing on lavatory walls.

**Observation** Intentional examination of something for the purpose of gathering facts.

**Obsessive–compulsive state** Recurrent mental event (thought, fear and impulse) which the patient cannot control, though he recognizes it to be morbid and irrational.

**Occupational cramps** Occurs in persons involved with complicated movements of the fingers for long periods of time, e.g. clerk, pianist, telegraphist and violinist.

**Occupational therapy** Therapeutic approach by means of purposeful occupation.

**Oculo-gyric crisis** Turning of the eyes in an upward direction. (*Syn.*, conjugate ocular spasm.)

**Oculomotor nerve** Third, motor nerve which supplies the muscles that move the eye.

**Oedipus complex** Desire of the son to displace his father and possess his mother.

**Olfactory nerve** First, sensory nerve concerned with the sense of smell

**Oligophrenia** Mental retardation.

**Oneiroid** Dream-like state.

**Oneirophrenia** Schizophrenia with a clouding of consciousness.

**Operant conditioning** Strengthening of a stimulus–response association by following the response with a reinforcing stimulus. (*Syn.* instrumental conditioning.)

**Ophthalmoplegia** Paralysis of eye movement.

**Opisthotonos** Backward arching of the whole body.

**Optic disc** Optic nerve leaving the eye, seen through an ophthalmoscope.

**Optic nerve** Second, sensory nerve concerned with vision.

**Organic** Pertaining to the parts of the body.

**Organic brain disease** Cerebral pathology with mental changes, as in pre-senile and senile dementias.

**Organization** Social group created to attain certain clearly defined goals.

**Organ neurosis** Psychosomatic disorder due to the actual or believed disorder of an organ.

**Orgasm** Sexual climax; moment of sudden release of tension.

**Orientation** Awareness of one's relationship to a person, place or time.

**Othello syndrome** Morbid sexual jealousy.

**Otorrhoea** Running from the ear.

**Over-flow incontinence** Constant dribbling due to over-distension of an insensitive bladder.

**Over-valued idea** Emotionally charged idea which tends to dominate the thought-processes.

**Ovum** Female sex cell. (*Pl.* ova.)

**Oxycephaly** Elongated head.

# P

**Palilalia**   Repetition of words with increasing speed and diminishing audibility. Occurs in post-encephalitis Parkinsonism.

**Palpitation**   Sensation of rapid beating of the heart; tachycardia.

**Panic**   Sudden feeling of terror. The principle signs and symptoms of acute anxiety or overwhelming dread are pallor, sweating, goose pimples, dry mouth, pupillary dilation, sinking feeling, frequency of micturition or defaecation, tachycardia and hyperventilation, resulting in a fight–flight reaction.

**Papez circuit**   Famous circuit described by Papez is:

Hippocampus → Hypothalamus

↑                    ↓

Cortex          ← Thalamus

This circuit is concerned with reactions related to emotions attaining awareness. The recticular system is connected to some of these structures as follows:

Reticular system → Hypothalamus

↓

Amygdala and Septal area

**Papilloedema**   Swelling of the optic nerve head (optic disc) as seen with an ophthalmoscope.

**Paramnesia**   Distortion or falsification of memory.

**Paranoia**   Psychosis characterized by fixed and systematized delusions, with a well-preserved personality and no hallucinations.

**Paranoid**   Reaction to feeling of persecution.

**Paranoid schizophrenia**   Delusions and hallucinations dominate the basic schizophrenic symptoms. (*Cf.* schizophrenia.)

**Paranoid states**   Unity of schizophrenia, paraphrenia and paranoia; delusionary states.

**Paraphasia**   Speech disorder in which the wrong word is used.

**Paraphrenia**   Characterized by unsystematized delusions associated with hallucinations. The personality is well preserved.

**Paraplegia**   Paralysis of both legs.

**Parasthesia**   Abnormal sensation in the skin, e.g. burning, tingling, 'pins and needles', in the absence of an external stimulus; and commonly due to irritation of the sensory pathway in the peripheral nerves or in the central nervous system.

**Pareidolia**   Illusion arising from ill-formed stimuli like clouds in the sky.

**Parkinson's disease**   Group of associated signs and symptoms resulting from disease of certain nerve cells situated at the base of the brain. There is muscular rigidity, tremor which increase on voluntary movement and inco-ordination. Muscles of the speech and face (mask-like face) may also be affected. This condition is also caused as a side-effect of drugs used in psychiatry. (*Syn.* paralysis agitans.)

**Passion**   Extremely intense and short-lived emotion.

**Passive**   Characterized by inactivity; submissive.

**Passivity feelings**   Actual feeling of being under some outside control, e.g. hypnosis. (*Syn.* delusions of influence.)

**Pathogenic**   Giving rise to disease or disorder.

**Pathognomonic**   Where certain features are characteristic of that disease.

**Pathological jealousy**   Certain degree of jealousy in a husband or wife may be normal, but if one is always suspecting the other of being unfaithful without any grounds for this, then it is morbid.

**Pathological lying**   *See* pseudologica phantastica.

## PERCEPTION

**Perception** Process of becoming aware of something through one of the senses, i.e. seeing, hearing, smelling, tasting or touching.

**Perceptual deprivation** Patient lies in a bed in a sound-proof room with translucent goggles, gloves and leggings. The effects of perceptual deprivation are: 1 affective change like fear, anxiety, even panic; 2 changes in perception, including negative after-images; 3 changes in perceptual motor skills; 4 over estimation of time; 5 changes in level of consciousness; 6 distractibility; 7 thought disorganization; 8 disturbance of body image; 9 sensitivity feelings of a paranoid character; and 10 somatic complaints. (*Syn.* sensory deprivation.)

**Performance tests** Psychological tests that rely on the ability to do things rather than tests based on language or symbols.

**Peripheral Neuritis** Bilateral and symmetrical affections of peripheral nerve-trunks, including both motor and sensory functions, first manifest at the distal part of the limbs.

**Perseveration** Tendency to keep repeating words, phrases, movement or behaviour, which is a common feature in organic mental syndromes. Thus, having replied correctly to a question, a patient may constantly repeat the answer instead of replying to further questions.

**Persona** Jung's personality mask or façade which is presented to the outside world.

**Personality** Sum total of an individual's behaviour.

**Personality disorders** Group of anomalies of personality which are not the result of a psychosis or psychoneurosis. This group includes paranoid, affective (cyclothymic), schizoid, explosive, anankastic (obsessive–compulsive), hysterical, asthenic and antisocial personality disorders. (*Syn.* psychopathic or sociopathic personalities.)

**Pes cavus** High arches of the feet.

**Petit mal** Sudden and transitory loss of consciousness starting during childhood. Classical three cycles per second (Hertz) spike and wave activity is seen in the EEG in this form of epilepsy. (*Syn.* absences; minor epilepsy.)

**Phantasy** Day dreaming.

**Phantom limb** Sensations that a limb is still present after its amputation.

**Phobia** Excessive or irrational fear of a particular object or situation. (*Cf.* Appendix D.)

**Phobic anxiety state** Morbid anxiety in the presence of an object or situation often amounting to panic.

**Pia mater** Innermost layer of meninges.

**Pick's disease** Progressive dementia with circumscribed cortical atrophy of fronto-temporal lobes.

**Pineal body** Structure lying in the centre of the skull, frequently calcified and visible on X-ray. (*Syn.* epiphysis cerebri.)

**Pituitary** Endocrine gland situated at the base of the skull.

**Plantar reflex** Toe movement on scratching the sole; it may be flexor or extensor. (L 1, S 1.)

**Plaques** Patches; usually applied to areas of demyelination in multiple sclerosis.

**Polarization** Group-specific mechanism in which complex emotional experiences become split into their component parts, thus to be seen more clearly at the opposite ends of the emotional spectrum or poles.

**Polioencephalitis** Brain stem infection by poliomyelitis virus.

**Polygraph** Instrument which measures the physiological changes that accompany emotional states, popularly called lie-detector.

**Porteus mazes** Test for foresight and impulsiveness. Subject has to trace out path through various mazes of increasing difficulty.

**Posterior horns**   Part of spinal grey matter receiving sensory roots.

**Preconscious**   That part of the mind between the unconscious and the conscious. Ideas from this part of the mind are not in awareness at any given moment but may be recalled. (Pcs).

**Prejudice**   Unreasonable attitudes with an emotional content based on false premises, either for or against something.

**Premenstrual tension**   Occurs during the second half of a menstrual cycle and consists of a number of physical and mental symptoms.

**Presenile dementia**   State of intellectual and/or emotional impairment due to organic cerebral changes occurring before the age of 65 years. Included in this category are: 1 Alzheimer's disease; 2 Pick's disease; 3 Creutzfeldt-Jakob's disease; and 4 Kraepelin's disease.

**Pressure cone**   Forcing of brain tissue through a foramen, as a result of high pressure from above, e.g. tentorial or cerebellar pressure cones.

**Primary delusion**   Delusion arising without any cause. Often the first sign of schizophrenia.

**Primary group**   Those groups with face-to-face association, of relative permanence, of relative intimacy, and a small number of persons involved; for example, the family, the neighbourhood. Psychotherapy group is a primary group; and secondary group lacks these features.

**Prodromal**   Early signs and symptoms of a disease.

**Programmed instruction**   Method of teaching based on operant conditioning in which correct responses are automatically reinforced, as for example, in a teaching machine.

**Projection**   Defence mechanism by which one judges others by one's self, e.g. to catch a thief is to set a thief. (*Opp*. introjection.)

**Propf schizophrenia** Schizophrenia occurring in the mentally subnormal. (*Syn.* grafted schizophrenia.)

**Proprioception** Sense of position and movement.

**Pseudocyesis** False pregnancy.

**Pseudodementia** *See* Ganser syndrome.

**Pseudohypertrophy** Apparent but not true enlargement.

**Pseudologia phantastica** Pathological lying is a substitute for a harsh repressive reality. Occurs in psychopathic disorders.

**Psyche** Greek goddess of soul; spirit; mind.

**Psychiatric social worker** Person who has done a course, sometimes a university degree in social science and has then further experience and training in social work with psychiatric patients and their families.

**Psychiatrist** Doctor with a basic medical degree and postgraduate training, experience and qualification in psychological medicine or psychiatry.

**Psychiatry** Branch of medicine dealing with mental illness.

**Psychic trauma** Mental or emotional shock.

**Psychoanalysis** Method of exploring the unconscious mind as devised by Sigmund Freud. It is not the analysis of the mind.

**Psychoanalyst** Layman, psychologist, clinical psychologist or psychiatrist who has undergone training analysis. A psychoanalyst is a psychotherapist.

**Psychobiology** Adolf Meyer's school of psychobiology which studies personality development in the light of environmental setting and the longitudinal growth.

**Psychodrama** Form of group therapy involving the dramatic staging of patient's signs and symptoms or problems by fellow patients or members of the therapeutic team.

**Psychodynamic**  Understanding and interpretation of psychiatric signs and symptoms or abnormal behaviour in terms of mental mechanisms, e.g. anxiety, a result of repressed aggression.

**Psychogalvanic response**  *See* Galvanic skin response (PGR).

**Psychogenic** ˙ Term applied to psychiatric illness in which the causes are largely psychological, arising from emotional difficulties within the individual and/or his reaction to external environment.

**Psychogram**  Graph to show the personality ratings of a person.

**Psychologist**  Graduate or post-graduate in psychology.

**Psychology**  Science of behaviour and experience.

**Psychomotor**  Motor activities initiated as a result of mental activity.

**Psychomotor acceleration**  Volubility and hyperactivity as seen in mania.

**Psychomotor retardation**  Slowing of speech and motor activity as seen in depression.

**Psychoneurosis**  *See* psychosis.

**Psychopathic disorder**  Means a persistent disorder or disability of mind (whether or not including subnormality of intelligence) which results in abnormally aggressive or seriously irresponsible conduct on the part of the patient, and requires or is susceptible to medical treatment. Cleckley in 1941 listed the following characteristics: 1 superficial charm and good intelligence; 2 absence of delusions and other signs of irrational thinking; 3 absence of nervousness or psychoneurotic manifestations; 4 unreliability; 5 untruthfulness. and insincerity; 6 lack of remorse or shame; 7 inadequately motivated antisocial behaviour; 8 poor judgment and failure to learn by experience; 9 pathological egocentricity and incapacity for love; 10 general poverty in major affective reactions; 11 specific loss of insight; 12 unresponsiveness in general interpersonal relations; 13 fantastic and un-invited behaviour with drink and sometimes without; 14 suicide rarely carried out; 15 sex life impersonal, trivial and poorly integrated; and 16 failure to follow any life plan.

**Psychopathology** Study of psychiatric signs and symptoms in terms of psychological processes involved.

**Psychosis and neurosis** Terms used to separate mental illnesses into two groups, the psychosis and the neurosis or psychoneurosis. The chief points of difference are:

| Points | Psychoneurosis | Psychosis |
|---|---|---|
| Delusion | Absent | Present |
| Environment | Distorted reaction to environment | Distorted view of environment |
| Hallucination | Absent | Present |
| Insight | Retained | Lost |
| Language | No disturbance | Disturbed |
| Personality | Partially involved | Wholly involved |
| Reaction | Partial | Total |
| Reality | Unchanged | Changed |
| Regression | Not so marked | Very marked |
| Sociability | Retained | Lost |
| Unconscious | Symbolically expressed | Verbally expressed |

Old dictum: When a patient does not realize that he is a patient he requires certification (compulsory detention).

**Psychosomatic disorders** Physical disorders which are aggravated or precipitated by emotional disturbances. Some of the psychosomatic disorders are: 1 respiratory disorders: a. asthma, b. vasomotor rhinitis, c. hay fever; 2 gastrointestinal disorders: a. peptic ulcer, b. colonic disorders; 3 skin disorders; 4 disorders of muscles and joints: a. rheumatoid arthritis, b. fibrositis; 5 endocrine disorders: a. hyperthyroidism, b. diabetes mellitus; 6 cardiovascular system: a. essential hypertension, b. coronary disease, c. cerebrovascular disease, d. migraine; and 7 disorders associated with menstrual and reproductive functions: a. amenorrhoea and oligomenorrhoea, b. dysmenorrhoea,

c. menorrhagia, d. pre-menstrual tension, and e. menopausal disturbances.

**Psychotherapy** Psychological methods of treatment of mental disorders.

**Ptosis** Drooping of the upper eye-lid.

**Puberty** Time of sexual maturity.

**Puerperal psychosis** Previously known as child-birth insanity. Begins acutely with transient clouding of consciousness. Depressive or schizophrenic and rarely manic features are seen. There is a risk of suicide or infanticide. This condition responds well to electroconvulsive therapy.

**Punch drunk** Boxer showing brain damage.

**Punishment** Sanction in criminal law is punitive. Today punishment is not regarded as the sole object of sanctions. Views are constantly changing. It has been held to be: compensation, deterrence, expiation, prevention, reformation and retribution.

**Pyknic physique** Kretschmer's short and stout type.

**Pyogenic** Causing the formation of pus.

**Pyramidal cells** Upper motor neurones.

**Pyramidal tract** Pathways controlling voluntary movement.

**Pyromania** Morbid compulsion to set fire to things.

# Q

**Q sort** Personality rating technique in which the subject sorts a large number of statements into piles which represent the degree to which he believes the statements apply to him.

**Quadriplegia**   Paralysis of all four limbs.

**Quasipsychotic state**   Hysterical pseudodementia or Ganser syndrome.

**Queckenstedt test**   Rise in lumbar CSF pressure on compressing the jugular vein.

# R

**Racial unconscious**   According to Carl Gustav Jung that part of the unconscious mind which derives from ancestral experience or function-engram. (*Syn.* collective unconscious; Rucs.)

**Rape**   Unlawful sexual intercourse with a woman without her consent by force, fear or fraud. It is an offence punishable with imprisonment to have sexual intercourse with a girl under 13 years, even with consent under 16 years and any age within prohibited degree of relationship (incest).

**Rapport**   Feeling of emotional contact with another person. (*Syn.* transference.)

**Rationalization**   Mental mechanism whereby ostensible reasons are devised to justify behaviour actually based on other motives.

**Raven's progressive matrices**   Non-verbal intelligence test. Subject has to complete abstract designs.

**Reaction**   Change in psychological state brought about by external events.

**Reaction formation**   Mental mechanism which keeps unconscious material from the conscious mind by presenting material opposite to the unconscious, e.g. sexual desire obscured by a prudish attitude.

**Reaction time**   Lapse of time between the application of a stimulus and its response.

**Reactive**  Term applied to depressive illness arising as a direct response of the patient to adverse external circumstances. (*Syn.* exogenous.)

**Recall**  Summon from memory a past experience; recollection.

**Receptor**  Special sensory nerve ending that receives stimuli.

**Recidivist**  Habitual criminal; persistent offender.

**Reciprocal inhibition**  Methods of inhibiting an anxiety response by eliciting a response incompatible with anxiety, e.g. systematic desensitization.

**Reflex**  Automatic and involuntary response to a stimulus.

**Registration**  Initial phase of memory process depending upon the faculties.

**Regression**  Reversion to a mode of behaviour and/or an emotional state appropriate to a younger age.

**Rehabitation**  Process of being restored to functioning as a fairly normal person, especially in respect to work and social life.

**Reinforcement**  Procedure which strengthens the frequency, speed or magnitude of a response.

**Repertory grid technique**  Method of assessing attitudes. Useful for investigating how a patient construes his illness.

**Repression**  Psychological process by which unacceptable impulses or ideas are rendered unconscious. In the individual, the repressed ideas may be translated and expressed as symptoms. In the group, cultural factors play a dynamic role in determining what is or is not acceptable and in moulding the nature of repression.

**Resignation**  Avoidance of any part of reality that brings inner conflicts into awareness.

**Resistance**  Instinctive opposition displayed towards any attempt to lay bare the unconscious.

**Response** Reaction by the organism.

**Retardation** Slow speech and behaviour, observed in depressive illness. All movements may be retarded and every action appears an extreme effort.

**Retention** Intermediate phase of the memory involving the consolidation of the enduring memory-trace or engram.

**Reticular formation** Groups of neurones found in the brain stem responsible for maintaining cortical excitation.

**Retirement** Major stress for men because there is loss of status, occupation and income.

**Retro-bulbar** Behind the eye.

**Rhinorrhoea** Running of the nose.

**Rigidity** Stiffness due to equal resistance in all muscles.

**Rinné test** Vibrating fork is placed over the mastoid process. When no longer heard it is held in front of the ear. Normally it is heard by air conduction after bone conduction ceases. In nerve deafness both are diminished, but air conduction remains better than bone conduction. In conduction deafness, bone conduction is better than air conduction. (*Cf.* Weber test.)

**Risus sardonicus** Semblance of a grin usually caused by spasm of the facial muscles.

**Ritual** System of ceremonies or procedures compulsively carried out without variation.

**Role playing** Function played by an individual in a group which may be primarily determined by the individual's attitudes, personality and previous roles, which he brings to the group; alternatively it may be the expression of the demands of the group as a whole.

**Romberg's sign** Patient stands upright with heels together without loss of balance whether the eyes are open or closed. But if the balance cannot be maintained after closing of the eyes, it is due to loss of postural sensation in the lower limbs. Occurs in tabes dorsalis; subacute combined degeneration.

**Roots**   Nerve fibres as they enter or leave the stem or cord.

**Rorschach diagnostic inkblots**   Projective test in which the subject has to interpret inkblot patterns. Used as an aid for the diagnosis of schizophrenia.

**Rorschach test**   Projection test in which the subject is asked to elaborate a series of ink blot patterns, some in colour.

**Rosenzweig picture frustration study**   Projective personality test. Consists of a number of pictures showing frustrating situations. The patient identifies himself with each situation.

**Rote learning**   Learning by repetition without regard to meaning or understanding.

**Rotter sentence completion test**   Projective personality test. Subject has to complete a form with unfinished sentences.

**Rud's syndrome**   Congenital ichthyosis with epilepsy and mental deficiency and occasionally spasticity.

# S

**Sadism**   Sexual perversion in which pleasure is obtained by inflicting pain.

**Salaam spasms**   Periodic and rhythmical movements of the head and the upper part of the body of about two seconds' duration with interval of about ten seconds which resemble a form of greeting.

**Satyriasis**   Excessive, pathological heterosexuality in the male; priapism. (*Opp.* nymphomania in female.)

**Scapegoating**   Process by which a recipient accepts the projections of others in the group. Sometimes there is an urgent need in the group to find a sacrificial victim to be punished, thereby avoiding more generalized violence, which might otherwise destroy the whole group.

**Schizoid type**  Shut-in, asocial type of personality.

**Schizophrenia**  'By the term dementia praecox or schizophrenia we designate a group of psychoses whose course is at times chronic, at times marked by intermittent attacks and which can stop or retrograde at any stage, but does not permit a full *restitutio ad integrum*. The disease is characterized by a specific type of thinking, feeling and relation to the external world which appears nowhere else in this particular disease' (Eugen Bleuler, 1911). It is a disharmony between the functions of the mind, like thinking, feeling and acting, e.g. the Queen of the world cheerfully sweeps the floor. The various forms of schizophrenia are: 1 simple, 2 hebephrenia, 3 catatonia, 4 paranoid, 5 schizo-affective and 6 pseudo-neurotic.

**Schnauzkrampf**  Exaggerated pouting or pursing protrusions of the lips. Characteristic of catatonic schizophrenia.

**Schonell's diagnostic attainment tests**  Achievement test for children of 8 to 14 years. A series of tests covering various aspects of English and mathematics.

**Sciatica**  Pain in the distribution of the sciatic nerve.

**Sclerosis**  Hardening.

**Scoptophilia**  Sexual excitement obtained from viewing sexual scenes; voyeurism; 'peeping Tom'.

**Scotoma**  Patch of blindness.

**Seizure**  Convulsion; fit.

**Sella turcica**  Saddle-shaped cavity at the base of the skull containing the pituitary gland.

**Sensation**  Experiencing a stimulus on a sensory nerve ending. A single sensation is a psychological myth. Multiple sensations are perception.

**Sensorium**   Inclusive term for all the special senses, e.g. the sensorium is clear.

**Sensory**   Concerned with sensation.

**Sensory deprivation**   *See* perceptual deprivation.

**Sentiment**   1 System of emotional organization centred around a particular object; 2 emotions are episodes in the life history of a sentiment.

**Set**   Readiness to perceive the environment in a particular way; tuning-in.

**Shaping**   Fashioning of new patterns of behaviour by reinforcing some responses and not reinforcing others.

**Sheldon's types**   Classification of personality types by physical build. Three main types are described: 1 endomorph, pyknic, reserved type; 2 ectomorph, asthenic, shut-in type; 3 mesomorph, athletic, energetic type. (*Syn.* somato types.)

**Shifting perception**   *See* figure-ground.

**Shoplifting**   Morbid desire to steal; kleptomania.

**Siblings**   Children of the same parents.

**Signe de magnan**   Tactile hallucinations. (*Cf.* formication.)

**Signe du miroir**   Pathognomonic of Alzheimer's disease. The patient sits in front of the mirror and talks to his own reflection as the memory of his personal identity is lost.

**Situation psychosis**   Psychosis arising from the individual's inability to cope with a difficult situation.

**Skill**   Ability to perform a complex act with precision.

**Skin potential**   Measurement of differences in electrical potential between an active and an inactive site on the skin.

**Skin resistance**   Measure of palmar sweating; galvanic skin response (GSR).

**Social**   Relating to the individual and his relationship with others of the same species.

**Social consciousness**   Being aware of one's relationships with the community.

**Social group**   Number of individuals collected together and having a common purpose.

**Social normal**   That which is accepted as normal by society at large.

**Social status**   Position of the individual within the social group.

**Sociology**   Scientific study of human society.

**Sociopath**   *See* personality disorder.

**Somatic**   Pertaining to the body.

**Somato types**   *See* Sheldon's types.

**Somnambulism**   Sleep walking; dissociated states that begin during sleep.

**Sopor**   State of drowsiness in which the patient can make some responses to stimuli.

**Space occupying lesion**   Tumour, or other growing lesion.

**Spastic**   Showing increased muscle tone. Patients suffering from cerebral palsy are sometimes referred to as 'spastics' because of the increased muscle tone.

**Spastic ataxia**   Combination of spasticity and unsteadiness.

**Speech disorders**   Disorganization of speech. Communication involves at least two persons. Disorders of speech are divided into: 1 amimia, absence of gestures; 2 aphonia, absence of sound or voice; and 3 agraphia, absence of pictorial symbols.

**Spinal-accessory nerve**   Eleventh, motor nerve consists of two portions: the cranial, supplying the pharynx and larynx; and the spinal, muscles of the neck.

**Spondylosis**   Degenerative changes in bones and discs in the spine.

**Spontaneous remission**  Recovery from illness, without any formal treatment.

**Stammering**  Irregular, often variable, hesitations, repetitions or blocking of certain speech sounds. (*Cf.* stuttering.)

**Startle reflex**  Complex universal response elicited by a loud and unexpected sound. A blink is followed by risus sardonicus and general crouching and shrinking of the body with slight flexion of the elbows and the knees.

**Statistics**  Branch of mathematics. A wide variety of methods are used for analysing, collecting, describing, interpreting, organizing and tabulating numerical data.

**Status epilepticus**  Recurrence without interruption of grand mal seizures in an epileptic.

**Stenosis**  Narrowing.

**Stereognosis**  Ability to identify objects by touch.

**Stereotaxis**  Accurately locating small lesions in the depths of the brain.

**Stereotypy**  Tendency to keep up mechanical repetition of some act, word or phrase.

**Stilted language**  Bombastic; pompous; not natural in manner.

**Stimulus**  This may be chemical, electrical, mechanical or thermal. (*Cf.* S → R.)

**Strabismus**  Squint.

**Strait-jacket**  Canvas shirt used to restrain violent psychotic patients; camisole.

**Stream of thought**  Continuity of thought.

**Stretch reflex**  Contraction of muscle following its sudden stretching.

**Stupor**  State of intense psychic inhibition during which regression may occur to an infantile level manifest by complete suppression of speech, movement and action. Stupor may be divided into: 1 psychogenic: catatonic, depressive, hysterical, manic and shock stupor; and 2 organic: dementia paralytica, drugs, encephalitis, epilepsy, pellagra, post-traumatic and tumours of frontal lobes and corpus callosum. (*Syn.* akinetic mutism.)

**Subacute** Applied to conditions which fall between acute and chronic in duration of illness.

**Subacute combined degeneration** Peripheral neuropathy with progressive degeneration of the posterior and lateral columns of the spinal cord. It is associated with vitamin $B_{12}$ deficiency.

**Subarachnoid** Between arachnoid and pia.

**Subarachnoid haemorrhage** Bleeding from a blood vessel underneath the arachnoid membrane, one of the coverings of the brain.

**Subdural** Between dura and arachnoid.

**Subdural haematoma** Accumulation of blood resulting from bleeding underneath the dura, a membrane covering the brain, superficial to the arachnoid. Subdural haemorrhage often develops slowly following a head injury.

**Sub-group** Splitting up of the group into smaller sections, which may lead to fragmentation or alternatively to consolidation for further development. (*Syn.* splinter group.)

**Subjective** Pertaining to the individual's own thoughts, feelings, actions or self.

**Sublimation** Process of transforming the energy of repressed conflicts and directing them to socially acceptable goals.

**Subnormality** Term applied to individuals unable to look after themselves adequately as a result of low intelligence.

**Suicide** Act of killing oneself; self-murder. An abortive attempt is often referred to as parasuicide. Not punishable now.

**Sulci** Furrows on the surface of the brain.

**Super-ego**  Part of the mental apparatus concerned with morality and self-criticism, partly conscious and partly unconscious. Loosely, the 'conscious' or moral code within the psyche.

**Superficial reflexes**  Polysynaptic response arising from the stimulation of superficial structures, e.g. abdominal, corneal and plantar reflexes.

**Supinator jerk**  Tap on the styloid process of the radius produces flexion of the elbow. (C 5, C 6.)

**Symbol**  1 That which figuratively represents something else; and 2 a sign that relies upon a convention accepted by its users, e.g. sign and symbol in communication.

**Symptomatic**  Representing a disease process.

**Symptom rating test**  Self-rating questionnaire in which the patient can indicate the number and severity of symptoms. Used to evaluate the effects of treatment.

**Syndrome**  Collection of signs and symptoms recurring frequently enough to be recognizable.

**Syphilis**  Veneral disease due to *Treponema pallidum*. In its later stages it can affect the central nervous system and cause dementia paralytica with characteristic neurological findings.

**Syringomyelia**  Cavities lying near the centre of the spinal cord filled with fluid and surrounded by glial tissue.

**Syrinx**  Cavity in brain-stem or cord.

**Systemic infection**  Infection affecting the body as a whole.

# T

**Tabes dorsalis**  Degeneration of first-order sensory neurones, central to the dorsal root ganglion, in the lower thoracic and lumbar nerve roots, as a sequel to syphilitic infection. Also known as loco-motor ataxia.

**Tavistock self-assessment inventory** Personality test covering various aspects based on factor analysis. Patient is required to agree or deny a series of statements.

**Taylor manifest anxiety scale** Questionnaire measuring anxiety.

**Tay–Sach's disease** *See* amaurotic family idiocy.

**Teaching machine** Instructional device which presents statements and questions in a careful step-by-step sequence, informing the learner of the correctness of his responses.

**Teichopsia** Flashes of light in migraine.

**Temperament** Individual's nature, especially the consistency of emotional reactions.

**Temporal lobe** One of the areas of the cortex of the brain. The temporal lobes are situated in the lower, lateral parts of each cerebral hemisphere.

**Temporal lobe epilepsy** Additional distinctive features are amnesia, automatism, altered consciousness and peculiar experiences of smell and taste. (*Syn.* psychomotor seizure.)

**Tension** Feeling of strain.

**Tentorial herniation** Forcing part of the brain through the tentorial hiatus.

**Tentorium** Tent-like sheet of dura separating cerebellum from cerebral hemispheres.

**Terman–Merril Stanford–Binet intelligence scale** Mental ability test of the verbal type. Popular test developed from original Binet–Simon test.

**Testamentary capacity** Sound disposing mind is required to make a valid Will. Mental disorder or compulsory detention in itself is no bar. Points to note are: 1 ability a. to realize the nature of the Will and its consequences, b. to recall the nature and extent of his property, and c. to recall the names of all near relatives; 2 absence: a. of a morbid state of mind, and b. of influence through fear, force or fraud. In case of doubt the testator should be re-examined. The beneficiary should not witness the Will.

**Test score**   Performance of a person in a test in relationship to the scale of normal scores.

**T-groups**   Stands for training groups in which awareness and verbalization of relationships and emotions are regarded as essential parts of learning process. (*Syn.* sensitivity or study groups.)

**Theca**   Space formed by the meninges containing CSF.

**Thematic apperception test**   Projective personality test. Consists of a series of pictures. (TAT.)

**Therapeutic community**   Main coined the phrase in 1946. It is the social organization in which a patient can derive benefit from being a member of it, through being part of the whole. Certain basic principles came to be evolved: democratization, permissiveness, communalism and finally reality-confrontation.

**Thinking**   Organization of mental powers into a course or series of ideas, usually initiated by a problem.

**Thought disorder**   Thinking is disordered in stream or content.

**Thyrotoxicosis**   Condition caused by overactivity of the thyroid gland. Hyperactivity, loss of weight and tremors are the classic signs and may be confused with a psychiatric disorder.

**Tics**   Involuntary spasmodic contractions of muscles, often repetitive and sometimes worse under stress. The movements are more stereotyped and repetitive than choreiform, e.g. a recurrent spasm in tic douloureux.

**Tinnitus**   Ringing in the ears.

**Todd's paralysis**   Temporary paralysis of a part following an epileptic fit.

**Token economy system**  Method of controlling the behaviour of a group of people in an institution, in which socialized, rational, adaptive behaviour is reinforced by tokens which can be exchanged for a variety of privileges. This has been applied to patients in the chronic wards of psychiatric hospitals.

**Tone**  Tension present in muscle at rest.

**Tonic**  Stage in convulsion during which the muscles are in sustained contraction.

**Topography**  Term used in psychoanalysis to describe the localization of the mind into the divisions of the super-ego, the ego and the id.

**Tracts**  Collection of nerve fibres having similar functions.

**Train of thought**  Flow of sequence of ideas.

**Trait**  Individual characteristic.

**Transference**  Projection of thoughts, feelings and wishes on to the others. Two different types of transference: 1 positive, predominantly libidinal, when the patient unrealistically overvalues or loves the analyst; and 2 negative, predominantly aggressive, when in reality the patient dislikes or hates the analyst without cause.

**Transsexualism**  Desire to change one's sex.

**Transvestism**  Wearing of clothes of the opposite sex to obtain sexual pleasure.

**Trauma**  Injury to the body or mind, the latter in the form of an emotional shock.

**Traumatic neurosis**  Psychoneurosis developing as the result of physical or psychological trauma.

**Trema**  German slang for stage fright before the performance begins. Suspiciousness, irritability and depression often characterize the prodromal period which is like an uneasy calm before the storm.

**Triceps jerk**  Tap on the triceps tendon of the flexed elbow results in the contraction of triceps. (C 6, C 7.)

**Trichotillomania**  Hair plucking is usually seen in young girls. It is a sign of serious emotional problem. Also occurs in mentally subnormal patients.

**Trigeminal nerve**  Fifth, mixed nerve consisting of a large sensory part with three sub-divisions: 1 ophthalmic, 2 maxillary, and 3 mandibular; and the motor part innervates the muscles of mastication.

**Trismus**  Spasmodic muscular contractions of the jaw muscles.

**Trisomy 21**  *See* Down's syndrome.

**Trochlear nerve**  Fourth, motor nerve which supplies the superior oblique muscle of the eye.

**Trombone tongue**  Forward and backward movements of the tongue resulting in slurred speech. Characteristic of dementia paralytica.

**Trophic**  Changes occurring in tissues which have lost their nerve supply.

**Trousseau's sign**  Pressure on the arm produces *main d'accoucheur* in latent tetany.

**Truancy**  Wilful avoidance of school.

**Tuberose sclerosis**  *See* epiloia.

**Turner's syndrome**  Chromosal abnormality with 45 chromosomes. Signs and symptoms include retardation in physical growth, ovarian dysgenesis and phenotypically to be female. Sex chromatin test is negative. (*Syn.* monosomy X.)

**Twilight state**  States of partial consciousness in which awareness seems limited, comprehension dulled and abnormal behaviour reflects the mental state.

# U

**Ulcerative colitis**   Disease with ulceration of the inner wall of the colon and rectum. It can be severe and persistent condition and sometimes leads to death.

**Unconscious**   Part of the mind not accessible to conscious thought; without consciousness or awareness (Ucs).

**Uniovular twins**   Identical twins with the same genetic make-up. Twins developed from a single ovum.

**Upper motor neurone**   Fibres arise from cells in the precentral gyrus (motor area). Opposite side of the body from below upwards is represented. Signs of a lesion of the upper motor neurone are: 1 loss of voluntary movement; 2 increase in muscle tone, spasticity; 3 reflexes: deep, increased; super-ficial, absent; 4 extensor plantar response; 5 no muscular atrophy; and 6 electrical reaction, unchanged.

# V

**Vaginismus**   Painful spasm of the vaginal muscles.

**Vagus nerve**   Tenth, mixed nerve receives afferent fibres from the pharynx, larynx, thoracic and abdominal viscera; and the efferent fibres innervate the thoracic and abdominal viscera.

**Ventilation**   Talking out of problems to relieve emotional tension.

**Ventricles**   Cavities in the brain containing CSF.

**Ventriculography**   The X-raying of the ventricles by injecting air directly into them.

**Verbigeration**   Morbid repetition of words, phrases and sentences.

**Vernon's test**   Mental ability test.

**Vertigo**   Sense of rotation.

**Vestibular**   Concerned with the labyrinth and its connections.

**Vibration sense**   Ability to appreciate vibrations when tuning fork, preferably of low frequency (128 Hz), is placed on the surface of the body. This is lost in tabes dorsalis, peripheral neuritis and normally in old age.

**Vineland social maturity scale**   Questionnaire to test social adjustment.

**Viral**   Due to infection by a virus.

**Vocational apperception test**   Designed to assess aptitude for different occupations (VAT).

**Volition**   Act of determining a course of action and of initiating it.

**Von Recklinghausen's disease**   Neurofibromatosis.

**Vorbeigehen**   Literally to walk past point; to pass over a subject silently, to reach beyond a significant point to another.

**Vorbeireden**   State of approximate answers to questions in Ganser's syndrome; to talk past point.

**Voyeurism**   Another name for 'peeping Tom'; scoptophilia.

# W

**WAIS**   Wechsler Adult Intelligence Scale. Mental ability test.

**WBIS**   Wechsler–Bellevue Intelligence Scale. Original test from which the WAIS was derived.

**Weber test**   Vibrating fork is placed on the midline of the skull. In conduction deafness the sound is heard better in the defective ear; in nerve deafness it seems louder in the normal ear. (*Cf.* Rinné test.)

**Wernicke's encephalopathy** Disorder consisting of vomiting, nystagmus, ophthalmoplegia, ataxia, disorientation, amnesia and coma occurring as a sequel to chronic alcoholism. Deficiency of vitamin $B_1$ is largely responsible for this condition which is also known as encephalitis haemorrhagica superior.

**White matter** Parts of brain and spinal cord containing myelinated fibres.

**Will** Legal document providing for the disposition of a person's property after his death, for which he must have a sound disposing mind; testamentary capacity.

**Wilson's disease** Dementia due to retention in the body of copper; hepatolenticular degeneration.

**WISC** Wechsler Intelligence Scale for Children. Test similar to the WAIS but for children.

**Withdrawal syndrome** Symptoms that appear in drug dependence patients when the drug is withdrawn.

**Witzelsucht** Facetiousness; seen in lesions of the frontal lobe of the brain.

**WMS** Wechsler Memory Scale. Test for recent and remote memories.

**Wonderland syndrome** Charles Lutwidge Dodgson, with the pen-name of Lewis Carroll, told stories to amuse Alice Liddell. Later these stories were published in *Alice's Adventures in Wonderland* (1865) and *Through the Looking-glass* (1871). Carroll suffered from classical migraine and projected the migrainous hallucinations into his stories. The manifestations of the wonderland syndrome can also be experienced by patients affected by hallucinogenic drugs, delirium tremens, schizophrenia and temporal lobe tumours.

**Word-salad** Incomprehensible speech containing nonsense syllables, jargons and neologism. Typical of schizophrenia.

# X

**Xanthopsia**   Yellow-sightedness.

**XYY**   Chromosomal abnormality in which an extra Y (male) chromosome is present. (Normal male has XY chromosome and normal female XX.) This occurs in about 4% of delinquents and criminals. XYY males are inclined to be tall, thin, myopic, backward, aggressive and sometimes even violent.

# Z

**Zahlenschreiben**   Ability to recognize numbers traced with a blunt object on the palm of the hand. Lost in lesions of the post-central (sensory) gyrus.

**Zollner illusion**   Illusion of visual space.

**Zung's depression scale**   Self-rating scale for depression or anxiety.

**Zygote**   Cell formed by the union of two gametes or sex cells. Zygotes are diploid and gametes are haploid.

# International Statistical Classification of Mental Disorders

### Section V of the International Statistical Classification of Diseases, Injuries and Causes of Death, 8th Revision 1965.

## *List of Four-digit Categories*

*Note.* Volume 1 of the International Classification shows 'inclusion terms' under each of these headings. It should be borne in mind that these include descriptions used in other parts of the world which are not in general use in this country.

### PSYCHOSES (290–299)

**290  Senile and pre-senile dementia**

    290.0   Senile dementia

    290.1   Pre-senile dementia

**291  Alcoholic psychosis**

    291.0   Delirium tremens

    291.1   Korsakov's psychosis (alcoholic)

    291.2   Other alcoholic hallucinosis

    291.3   Alcoholic paranoia

    291.9   Other and unspecified

**292  Psychosis associated with intracranial infection**

    292.0   With general paralysis

    292.1   With other syphilis of central nervous system

    292.2   With epidemic encephalitis

    292.3   With other and unspecified encephalitis

    292.9   With other and unspecified intracranial infection

### 293 Psychosis associated with other cerebral condition

293.0 With cerebral arteriosclerosis
293.1 With other cerebrovascular disturbances
293.2 With epilepsy
293.3 With intracranial neoplasm
293.4 With degenerative diseases of the central nervous system
293.5 With brain trauma
293.9 With other and unspecified cerebral condition

### 294 Psychosis associated with other physical condition

294.0 With endocrine disorders
294.1 With metabolic and nutritional disorders
294.2 With systemic infections
294.3 With drug or poison intoxication
294.4 With childbirth
294.8 With other physical conditions
294.9 With unspecified physical condition

### 295 Schizophrenia

295.0 Simple type
295.1 Hebephrenic type
295.2 Catatonic type
295.3 Paranoid type
295.4 Acute schizophrenic episode
295.5 Latent schizophrenia
295.6 Residual schizophrenia
295.7 Schizo-affective type
295.8 Other
295.9 Unspecified type

### 296 Affective psychoses

296.0 Involutional melancholia
296.1 Manic-depressive psychosis, manic type
296.2 Manic-depressive psychosis, depressed type
296.3 Manic-depressive psychosis, circular type
296.8 Other
296.9 Unspecified

## 297 Paranoid states
297.0   Paranoia
297.1   Involutional paraphrenia
297.9   Other

## 298 Other psychoses
298.0   Reactive depressive psychosis
298.1   Reactive excitation
298.2   Reactive confusion
298.3   Acute paranoid reaction
298.9   Reactive psychosis unspecified

## 299 Unspecified psychosis

# NEUROSES, PERSONALITY DISORDERS AND OTHER NON-PSYCHOTIC MENTAL DISORDERS (300–309)

## 300 Neuroses
300.0   Anxiety neurosis
300.1   Hysterical neurosis
300.2   Phobic neurosis
300.3   Obsessive compulsive neurosis
300.4   Depressive neurosis
300.5   Neurasthenia
300.6   Depersonalization syndrome
300.7   Hypochondriacal neurosis
300.8   Other
300.9   Unspecified neurosis

## 301 Personality disorders
301.0   Paranoid
301.1   Affective
301.2   Schizoid
301.3   Explosive
301.4   Anankastic
301.5   Hysterical

301.6 Asthenic
301.7 Antisocial
301.8 Other
301.9 Unspecified

## 302 Sexual deviation

302.0 Homosexuality
302.1 Fetishism
302.2 Paedophilia
302.3 Transvestitism
302.4 Exhibitionism
302.8 Other
302.9 Unspecified

## 303 Alcoholism

303.0 Episodic excessive drinking
303.1 Habitual excessive drinking
303.2 Alcoholic addiction
303.9 Other and unspecified alcoholism

## 304 Drug dependence

304.0 Opium, opium alkaloids and their derivatives
304.1 Synthetic analgesics with morphine-like effects
304.2 Barbiturates
304.3 Other hypnotics and sedatives or tranquillizers
304.4 Cocaine
304.5 Cannabis sativa
304.6 Other psycho-stimulants
304.7 Hallucinogenics
304.8 Other
304.9 · Unspecified

## 305 Physical disorders of presumably psychogenic origin

305.0 Skin
305.1 Musculo-skeletal
305.2 Respiratory

305.3   Cardiovascular
305.4   Haemic and lymphatic
305.5   Gastro-intestinal
305.6   Genito-urinary
305.7   Endocrine
305.8   Organs of special sense
305.9   Other

## 306   Special symptoms not elsewhere classified

306.0   Stammering and stuttering
306.1   Specific learning disturbance
306.2   Tics
306.3   Other psychomotor disorders
306.4   Specific disorders of sleep
306.5   Feeding disturbances
306.6   Enuresis
306.7   Encopresis
306.8   Cephalalgia
306.9   Other

## 307   Transient situational disturbances

## 308   Behaviour disorders of childhood

## 309   Mental disorders not specified as psychotic associated with physical conditions

309.0   With intracranial infections
309.1   With drug, poison or systemic intoxication
309.2   With brain trauma
309.3   With circulatory disturbance
309.4   With epilepsy
309.5   With disturbance of metabolism, growth or nutrition
309.6   With senile or pre-senile brain disease
309.7   With intracranial neoplasm
309.8   With degenerative diseases of central nervous system
309.9   With other or unspecified physical condition

## MENTAL RETARDATION (310–315)

The following four-digit sub-division may be used with categories (310–315):

    .0   Following infections and intoxications
    .1   Following trauma or physical agents
    .2   With disorders of metabolism, growth or nutrition
    .3   Associated with gross brain disease (postnatal)
    .4   Associated with diseases and conditions due to (unknown) prenatal influence
    .5   With chromosomal abnormalities
    .6   Associated with prematurity
    .7   Following major psychiatric disorder
    .8   With psycho-social (environmental) deprivation
    .9   Other and unspecified

**310  Borderline mental retardation**

**311  Mild mental retardation**

**312  Moderate mental retardation**

**313  Severe mental retardation**

**314  Profound mental retardation**

**315  Unspecified mental retardation**

# APPENDIX B

# List of Abbreviations

| | | | | |
|---|---|---|---|---|
| AA | . | . | . | Alcoholics Anonymous |
| ANS | . | . | . | Autonomic nervous system |
| CA | . | . | . | Chronological age |
| CNS | . | . | . | Central nervous system |
| Cps | . | . | . | Cycles per second (*Syn.* Hz) |
| CR | . | . | . | Conditioned response |
| CS | . | . | . | Conditioned stimulus |
| Cs | . | . | . | Conscious |
| CSF | . | . | . | Cerebrospinal fluid |
| E | . | . | . | Experimenter (*Pl.* Es) |
| EA | . | . | . | Educational age |
| ECG | . | . | . | Electrocardiogram (*Syn.* EKG) |
| ECoG | . | . | . | Electrocorticogram |
| ECT | . | . | . | Electroconvulsive therapy (*Syn.* EST) |
| EEG | . | . | . | Electroencephalogram |
| EKG | . | . | . | Electrocardiogram (*Syn.* ECG) |
| EMG | . | . | . | Electromyogram |
| EPI | . | . | . | Eysenck personality inventory |
| ESP | . | . | . | Extrasensory perception |
| EST | . | . | . | Electric shock therapy (*Syn.* ECT) |
| f | . | . | . | Frequency |
| GBH | . | . | . | Grievous bodily harm |
| Gp | . | . | . | Group |
| GPI | . | . | . | General paralysis of the insane |
| GSR | . | . | . | Galvanic skin response (*Cf.* PGR) |
| Hz | . | . | . | Hertz (*Syn.* Cps) |
| IQ | . | . | . | Intelligence quotient |
| LP | . | . | . | Lumbar puncture |
| M | . | . | . | Arithmetic mean |
| MA | . | . | . | Mental age |
| Mdn | . | . | . | Median |
| MHA | . | . | . | Mental Health Act |
| MMPI | . | . | . | Minnesota multiphasic personality inventory |

| | | | | | |
|---|---|---|---|---|---|
| Mo | . | . | . | . | Mode |
| n | . | . | . | . | Number of cases |
| NS | . | . | . | . | Nervous system |
| O | . | . | . | . | Observer |
| OT | . | . | . | . | Occupational therapy |
| p | . | . | . | . | Percentile |
| Pcs | . | . | . | . | Preconscious |
| PGR | . | . | . | Psychogalvanic response (*Cf*. GSR) |
| R | . | . | . | . | Response |
| *r* | . | . | . | . | Product–moment correlation coefficient |
| RAS | . | . | . | Reticular activating system |
| RT | . | . | . | . | Reaction time |
| Rucs | . | . | . | Racial unconscious |
| S | . | . | . | . | 1 Stimulus; 2 subject (*Pl*. Ss) |
| s | . | . | . | . | Sensation |
| SD | . | . | . | . | Standard deviation |
| SOR | . | . | . | Stimulus–organism-response |
| SR | . | . | . | . | Stimulus-response |
| *t* | . | . | . | . | Ratio of any statistic to the standard error |
| TAT | . | . | . | Thematic apperception test |
| TE | . | . | . | . | Trial and error |
| Ucs | . | . | . | . | Unconscious |
| UCR | . | . | . | Unconditioned response |
| UCS | . | . | . | Unconditioned stimulus |
| *v* | . | . | . | . | Coefficient of variation |
| VAT | . | . | . | Vocational apperception test |
| WAIS | . | . | . | Wechsler adult intelligence scale |
| WMS | . | . | . | Wechsler memory scale |
| X | . | . | . | . | 1 Female chromosome; 2 raw score |
| *x* | . | . | . | . | Deviation of a class interval from a mean |
| Y | . | . | . | . | 1 Dependent variable; 2 male chromosome |
| *y* | . | . | . | . | Value of an ordinate |
| Z | . | . | . | . | Standard score |

# APPENDIX C

# A guide to
# Prefixes and Suffixes

| P or S | Meaning | Example |
|---|---|---|
| a- | absence | amentia; amnesia |
| ab- | away from | abnormal; abient |
| acro- | height | acrophobia |
| acou- | to hear | acoustics |
| ad- | to; toward | adrenal; adient |
| alb- | white | albino |
| ambi- | both | ambivalent |
| an- | without | anosmia |
| ana- | up | analysis |
| ante- | before | antenatal |
| antero- | in front of | anterograde |
| anthropo- | man | anthropology |
| anti- | against | antidepressant |
| arach- | spider | arachnoid |
| audio- | hearing | audiology |
| auri- | ear | auriscope |
| auto- | self | automatic; autosome |
| bi- | two | bisexual; bivalent |
| bas- | a step | a-basia |
| bio- | life | biology |
| cata- | down; low | catalepsy; catatonia |
| -cele | a rupture | hydrocele |
| cephalo- | brain; head | en-cephalitis |
| cerebro- | brain | cerebrospinal |
| chir- | hand-work | chirurgeon (surgeon) |
| chor- | a dance | chorea |
| chrom- | colour | chromosome |
| -cide | kill | homicide; suicide |
| claus- | shut in | claustrophobia |
| contra- | against | contraindication |
| corp- | body | corpse |

| P or S | Meaning | Example |
|--------|---------|---------|
| crem- . | crime . . . . | criminology |
| cyc- . . | circular . . . . | cyclothymia |
| di- . . | two . . . . . | dichromatic |
| dia- . . | across; between . | diaphragm |
| dis- . . | separate. . . . | disorientation; dissociation |
| dys- . . | impaired; morbid . | dyscalculia |
| echo- . | repetition . . . | echolalia |
| ecto- . . | outer . . . . | ectoderm |
| endo- . | inner . . . . | endoderm; endogenous |
| enter- . | piece of gut . . . | dysentery |
| epi- . . | above . . . . | epidermis |
| erg- . . | work . . . . | ergomania |
| -esthesia . | sensitivity . . . | synaesthesia |
| eti- . . | cause . . . . | aetiology |
| ex- . . | out of . . . . | explosive |
| exo- . . | outer . . . . | exogenous |
| extero- . | from outside . . | exteroceptor |
| fis- . . | split . . . . . | fissure |
| flag- . . | whip . . . . | flagellation |
| -flu- . . | to flow . . . . | con-flu-ence; in-flu-enza |
| fra- . . | break into pieces . | fracture; fragmentation |
| -genetic . | to do with origins . | phylogenetic |
| gli- . . | glue . . . . . | neuroglia |
| gno- . . | to know . . . . | a-gno-sia |
| -gram- . | is written . . . | electroencephalogram |
| -graph- . | to write . . . . | graphospasm (writer's cramp) |
| gyn- . . | woman . . . . | gynaecology |
| hebe- . | youth . . . . | hebephrenia |
| hema- . | blood . . . . | haematology |
| hemi- . | half . . . . . | hemiplegia |
| herm- . | androgyne; bisexual | hermaphrodite |
| hern- . | a rupture . . . | hernia |
| hetero- . | different . . . | heterosexual |
| hipp- . | horse . . . . | hippocampus |
| homo- . | similar . . . . | homosexual |
| hydr- . | water . . . . | hydrocephalus |

| P *or* S | | *Meaning* | | *Example* |
|---|---|---|---|---|
| hyper- | . | above; increase | . | hypertension |
| hypno- | . | sleep . . . | . | hypnosis |
| hypo- | . | below; decrease | . | hypotension |
| hyst- | . | womb . . . | . | hysteria |
| -ia | . | condition . . | . | phobia |
| -ian | . | pertaining to . | . | Pavlovian |
| iatro- | . | medicine; healing | . | iatrogenic |
| -iatry | . | cure . . . . | . | psychiatry |
| -ical | . | pertaining to . | . | neurological |
| ichthyo- | . | fish . . . . | . | ichthyosis |
| -ictal | . | stroke; seizure . | . | post-ictal |
| ictero- | . | yellow; jaundice | . | icterogenic |
| ideo | . | thought . . . | . | ideology |
| idio- | . | one's own . . | . | idiopathic |
| infra- | . | below . . . | . | infraclavicular |
| injecto- | . | throw in . . | . | injection |
| inter- | . | between . . . | . | inter-vertebral |
| intero- | . | from inside . . | . | interoceptor |
| intra- | . | from within . | . | intracerebral |
| intro- | . | directed inward | . | introvert |
| irid- | . | iris . . . . | . | iridectomy |
| -ism | . | doctrine; theory | . | invalidism |
| iso- | . | equal . . . | . | isomer |
| -ist | . | to practice . . | . | alienist (psychiatrist) |
| kine- | . | movement . . | . | kinesthesia |
| -lalia | . | talk . . . . | . | echolalia |
| -leps | . | seizure . . . | . | epilepsy |
| -logos | . | discourse . . | . | psychology |
| -lys | . | break up . . | . | psychoanalysis |
| macro- | . | large . . . | . | macrocephaly |
| mal- | . | bad . . . . | . | malaria |
| -mani- | . | madness . . | . | mania; kleptomania |
| manu- | . | hand . . . | . | manipulation |
| mel- | . | honey . . . | . | mellitus |
| mens- | . | periods . . . | . | menses |
| meso- | . | middle . . . . | . | mesoderm |

| P or S | Meaning | Example |
|--------|---------|---------|
| meta- | beyond | metapsychology |
| micro- | small | microcephaly |
| -mnes | mind | dysmnesia |
| mono- | single | monovalent |
| morb- | disease | morbid |
| morph- | form | morphology |
| -mot- | motion | emotion |
| multi- | many | multipolar |
| musc- | a fly | mosquito |
| my- | muscle | myasthenia |
| myel- | pith | myelin |
| neo- | recent | neo-Darwinism |
| nomen- | name | nomenclature |
| non- | not | non-viable |
| nycto- | night | nyctophobia |
| nymph- | a woman | nymphomania |
| oculo- | eye | oculomotor |
| -oid | likeness | paranoid |
| -oma | a growth | neuroma |
| omni- | all | omnipotent |
| onto- | existence | ontology |
| oph- | the eye | ophthalmia |
| -opia | vision | myopia |
| ortho- | correct | orthodox |
| -osis | disease | psychoneurosis |
| -osmia | smell | anosmia |
| oto- | ear | otology |
| ov- | egg | ovum |
| pan- | all | panacea |
| para- | abnormal; beside | paranoia |
| ped- | child | paediatrician |
| peri- | around | periphery |
| phas- | saying | aphasia |
| -philia | love | agoraphilia |
| -phobia | fear | claustrophobia |
| phren- | mind | hebephrenia |

| P or S | Meaning | Example |
|--------|---------|---------|
| phylo- . | race . . . . . | phylogenetic |
| pneumo- | air . . . . . | bronchopneumonia |
| post- . . | after . . . . . | post-mortem |
| pre- . . | in front . . . . | prefrontal |
| pro- . . | before . . . . | prognosis |
| pseudo- . | false . . . . . | pseudocyesis |
| psycho- . | mind . . . . | psychosurgery |
| pyr- . . | fire . . . . . | pyromania |
| quadri- . | four . . . . . | quadriplegia |
| rhe- . . | to flow . . . . | amenorrhoea |
| retro- . | behind . . . . | retroactive |
| schi- . . | to split . . . . | schizophrenia |
| scler- . | hardness . . . | arteriosclerosis |
| -scope . | viewing . . . . | stroboscope |
| scoto- . | darkness . . . | scotoma |
| semi- . | half . . . . | semiconscious |
| socio- . | companion . . . | sociology |
| -som- . | body . . . . | psychosomatic |
| stereo- . | solid . . . . . | stereoscope |
| -sthen- . | strength . . . . | neurasthenia |
| stig- . . | a mark . . . . | stigmata |
| sub- . . | below . . . . | subconscious |
| super- . | above . . . . | superfecundation |
| supra- . | on top of . . . | supraclavicular |
| sym- . . | with . . . . . | sympathy |
| syn- . . | together . . . . | syndrome |
| syri- . . | a pipe . . . . | syringomyelia |
| tach- . | fast . . . . . | tachycardia |
| tele- . . | distant . . . . | telepathy |
| -ther- . | to treat . . . . | psychotherapy |
| thym- . | mind . . . . | cyclothymia |
| -tomy- . | cut . . . . . | leucotomy |
| tort- . . | twist . . . . . | torticollis |
| -troph- . | nourishment . . | dystrophy |
| trans- . | across . . . . | transference |
| trich- . | hair . . . . . | trichotillomania |

| P or S | Meaning | Example |
|--------|---------|---------|
| -typ- | form; type | stereotypy |
| ultra- | beyond | ultravirus |
| un- | not | unconscious |
| uni- | one | univalent |
| -vert- | to turn | vertigo |
| xan- | yellow | xanthopsia |
| xen- | stranger | xenophobia |
| xero- | dry | xerophagia |
| zoo- | animal | zoopsia |

Increase your vocabulary by simple mental exercise! The following example is a combination of the prefixes and suffixes of the root-word 'pathos' meaning 'suffering':

| | | |
|---|---|---|
| antipathy | idiopathic | allopathy |
| apathy | pathognomonic | homeopathy |
| empathy | pathological | hydropathy |
| sympathy | psychopathological | osteopathy |

# APPENDIX D

# Common Phobias

| | |
|---|---|
| Air . . . . . . . | aerophobia |
| Animals . . . . . . | zoophobia |
| Bacteria . . . . . . | bacteriophobia |
| Bees . . . . . . | apiphobia |
| Blood . . . . . . | haematophobia |
| Blushing . . . . . | ereuthophobia |
| Cancer . . . . . . | cancerophobia |
| Cats . . . . . . | gatophobia |
| Choking . . . . . . | pnigophobia |
| Closed space . . . . | claustrophobia |
| Corpse . . . . . . | necrophobia |
| Death . . . . . . | thanatophobia |
| Dirt . . . . . . | mysophobia |
| Disease . . . . . . | pathophobia |
| Dogs . . . . . . | cynophobia |
| Drinking . . . . . | dipsophobia |
| Electricity . . . . . | electrophobia |
| Fire . . . . . . | pyrophobia |
| God . . . . . . | theophobia |
| Grave . . . . . . | taphophobia |
| Heights . . . . . . | acrophobia |
| Marriage . . . . . | gamophobia |
| Men . . . . . . | androphobia |
| Night . . . . . . | nyctophobia |
| Open space . . . . . | agoraphobia |
| Poisoning . . . . . | toxicophobia |
| Pregnancy . . . . . | maieusiophobia |
| Ridicule . . . . . . | catagelophobia |
| Self . . . . . . | autophobia |
| Sex act . . . . . . | coitophobia |
| Sin . . . . . . | hamartophobia |
| Snakes . . . . . . | ophidiophobia |
| Spiders . . . . . . | arachneophobia |

| | | |
|---|---|---|
| Stealing . . . . . . . | kleptophobia |
| Strangers . . . . . | xenophobia |
| Water . . . . . . | hydrophobia |
| Women . . . . . . | gynaephobia |
| Work . . . . . . | ergophobia |

Substitute 'philia' (love) for 'phobia' (fear).

# Normal Values in the Body

*Blood*

| | |
|---|---|
| Alkaline reserve . . . . . | 53–77 ml $CO_2$/dl plasma |
| Bilirubin (serum) . . . . . | 0.2–0.8 mg/dl |
| Calcium (serum): | |
| non-diffusible . . . . . | 4–5 mg/dl |
| diffusible . . . . . . | 5–6.5 mg/dl |
| | 2.5–3.25 mmol/litre |
| Cholesterol: | |
| esterified in plasma . . . . | $128 \pm 23$ mg/dl |
| esterified in corpuscles . . | $9 \pm 6$ mg/dl |
| free in plasma . . . . | $53 \pm 22$ mg/dl |
| free in corpuscles . . . | $130 \pm 30$ mg/dl |
| Mean corpuscular haemoglobin . | $29 \pm 2$ $\mu$g |
| Packed cell volume: | |
| male . . . . . . . | 40–54 per cent |
| female . . . . . . | 36–47 per cent |
| Mean corpuscular volume . . | $87 \pm \mu m^3$ |
| Mean corpuscular haemoglobin | |
| concentration . . . . | $34 \pm 2$ per cent |
| Plasma electrolytes: | |
| calcium . . . . . . | 2.4–2.8 mmol/litre |
| chloride . . . . . . | 101–106 mmol/litre |
| potassium . . . . . | 3.9–5 mmol/litre |
| sodium . . . . . . | 137–148 mmol/litre |
| Circulation time: | |
| arm to tongue . . . . | 9–16 seconds |
| arm to lung . . . . . | 3.5–8 seconds |
| Coagulation time: | |
| capillary . . . . . . | 10–15 min at room temp |
| venous . . . . . . | 3–7 min at 37°C |
| Haemoglobin: | |
| male . . . . . . . | $16 \pm 2$ g/dl blood |
| female . . . . . . | $14 \pm 2$ g/dl blood |

pH . . . . . . . . . 7.3–7.5
Red blood cells:
   male . . . . . . . . 5.4 ± 0.8 millions/mm³
   female . . . . . . 4.8 ± 0.6 millions/mm³
Plasma folate . . . . . 5.9–21 ng/dl
Plasma vitamin $B_{12}$ . . . . 106–925 pg/dl
Plasma iron. . . . . . 50–175 μg/dl
Plasma iron-binding capacity. . 300–360 μg/dl
Protein-bound iodine . . . 4–8 μg/dl
White blood cells mm³. . . 5000–10,000
   neutrophils:
      juvenile . . . . . 3–5 per cent. 150–400
      segmented. . . . . 54–62 per cent 3000–5800
    eosinophils . . . . . 1–3 per cent 50–250
    basophils . . . . . . 0–0.75 per cent 15–50
    lymphocytes . . . . . 25–33 per cent 1500–3000
    monocytes . . . . . 3–7 per cent 285–500
Glucose:
   fasting . . . . . . 60–120 mg/dl
   normal . . . . . . 180 mg/dl
Platelets. . . . . . . 150,000–500,000 mm³
Sedimentation rate:
   male . . . . . . . 1 h: 3–5 mm
                         2 h: 7–15 mm
   female . . . . . . 1 h: 7–12 mm
                         2 h: 12–17 mm
Urea:
   male . . . . . . . 26–46 mg/dl
   female . . . . . . 11–29 mg/dl
Uric acid . . . . . . 1–5 mg/dl
Volume of whole blood:
   male . . . . . . . 75.5 dl/kg
   female . . . . . . 66.5 dl/kg

*Cerebrospinal fluid*
  Appearance. . . . . . . clear and colourless
  Lymphocytes . . . . . . 0–4/mm³

Electrolytes:
  calcium . . . . . . . 2.2–2.6 mmol/litre
  chloride . . . . . . . 120–128 mmol/litre
  potassium . . . . . . 2.4–3.2 mmol/litre
  sodium . . . . . . . 140–150 mmol/litre
Glucose . . . . . . . . 45–100 mg/dl
Pressure . . . . . . . . 100–130 mm
Protein:
  total . . . . . . . . 12–43 mg/dl
  albumin . . . . . . . 40–70 per cent
  globin . . . . . . . 25–60 per cent
Urea . . . . . . . . 8–40 mg/dl
Lange curve:
  paretic . . . . . . . . 5555432100
  leutic . . . . . . . . 0123210000
  meningitic . . . . . . 0001344310

*Gastric secretion*
Fasting volume . . . . . . 50–100 ml
pH . . . . . . . . 0.9–1.5
Acid:
  total . . . . . . . . 10–15 mmol/litre
  free . . . . . . . . 0–50 mmol/litre

*Urine*
Reaction . . . . . . . pH 4.8–7.4
Specific gravity . . . . . . 1.01–1.025
Volume . . . . . . . . 8–20 dl in 24 h
Electrolytes:
  calcium . . . . . . . 2–23 mmol in 24 h
  chloride . . . . . . . 58–250 mmol in 24 h
  potassium . . . . . . 53–91 mmol in 24 h
  sodium . . . . . . . 40–156 mmol in 24 h
  17-ketosteroids:
    male . . . . . . . 10–30 mg in 24 h
    female . . . . . . . 5–14 mg in 24 h
Urea . . . . . . . . 15–35 g in 24 h

*Faeces*

| | |
|---|---|
| Total fat . . . . . . . | 10–20 per cent w/w |
| free fatty acid . . . . . | 7.5–15 per cent w/w |
| neutral fat . . . . . . | 2.5–5 per cent w/w |

# **APPENDIX F**

# Essential Statistical Formulae

1 $M = \dfrac{\Sigma \chi}{N}$  for ungrouped data.

2 $M = AM + \left(\dfrac{\Sigma \chi}{N}\right) i$  for grouped data.

3 $Mdn = 1 + i\left(\dfrac{\frac{1}{2}N - F}{fp}\right)$ calculated from below up, grouped data.

4 $SD \text{ or } \sigma = \sqrt{\left(\dfrac{\Sigma \chi^2}{N}\right)}$  for ungrouped data.

5 $SD \text{ or } \sigma = \sqrt{\left(\dfrac{\Sigma f \chi^2}{N}\right)}$  for grouped data.

6 $PE = 0.6745\sigma$  probable error.

7 $P = 1 + \left(\dfrac{pN - F}{fp}\right) i$  percentile.

8 $Z = 50 + 10\dfrac{X - M}{\sigma}$  Z score.

9 $y = \dfrac{N}{\sigma \sqrt{\pi^2}} e^{\frac{\chi^2 2}{2\sigma}}$  Normal probability curve.

10 $V = \dfrac{100\sigma}{N}$  Coefficient of variation.

11    $r = \dfrac{\Sigma xy}{N\sigma x\sigma y}$        Pearson product—moment coefficient of correlation.

12    $\sigma_r = \dfrac{1}{\sqrt{(N-1)}}$        Standard error of Pearson correlation.

13    $byx = r\dfrac{\sigma y}{\sigma x}, \quad bxy = r\dfrac{\sigma x}{\sigma y}$        Regression coefficients.

14    $t = \dfrac{M_1 - M_2}{\sigma d_{1-2}}$        $t$ ratio.

15    $\sigma^2 = \dfrac{\Sigma x^2}{N}$        Variance.

16    $\chi^2 = \dfrac{\Sigma(f_o - f_e)^2}{fe}$        Chi square.

## APPENDIX H

# Essentials

of the

# Mental Health Act, 1959

Received the Royal Assent on 29 July, 1959, and came into effect on 1 November, 1960.

———

Contains IX parts, 154 sections and eight schedules.

———

## MAIN PRINCIPLES

The underlying principles are:

1  That treatment, in hospital and outside, should be given on voluntary or informal basis;

2  That compulsory admission, in the interest of the patient or the society, should be for a limited period; and

3  That emphasis should be shifted from institutional care to community care.

## Part I  S 1–3

### Introduction

All previous legislation dealing with mental illness and mental deficiency is repealed and one Act is substituted. The Board of Control is dissolved. A Mental Health Review Tribunal to be set up for each Regional Hospital Board.

## PART I  S 4 (1–4)

### Definitions

Mental disorder means mental illness, arrested or incomplete development of mind, psychopathic disorder and any other disorder or disability of mind.

Severe subnormality means a state of arrested or incomplete development of mind, which includes subnormality of intelligence, and is of such a nature or degree that the patient is incapable of living an independent life or of guarding himself against serious exploitation, or will be so incapable when of an age to do so.

Subnormality means a state of arrested or incomplete development of mind (not amounting to severe subnormality), which includes subnormality of intelligence, and is of a nature or degree which requires or is susceptible to medical treatment or other special care or training of the patient.

Psychopathic disorder means a persistent disorder or disability of mind (whether or not including subnormality of intelligence) which results in abnormally aggressive or seriously irresponsible conduct on the part of the patient, and requires or is susceptible to medical treatment.

## PART I  S 5 (1–2)

### Informal admission

Patient who requires treatment for mental disorder may be admitted to any hospital or mental nursing home without formality.

An infant who has attained the age of 16 years and is capable of expressing his own wishes may be admitted informally, notwithstanding the right of custody or control vested by law in the parent or guardian.

## PART II  S 6–13

### Local Authority services

The provision and maintenance of residential accommodation, training centres, appointment of mental welfare officers, supervision of persons placed under guardianship and ancillary or supplementary services.

## PART III   S 14–24

### Registration of homes
Registration of mental nursing homes and residential homes.

## PART IV   S 25–35

### Compulsory admission
Procedures for hospitalization under Sections 25, 26, 29 and 30 (2) and for guardianship under Section 33:

## Section 25    Admission for observation

| | |
|---|---|
| *Applicant* | (a) Nearest relative<br>or<br>(b) Mental Welfare Officer    Form 1. Must see the patient personally within 14 days of date of application. |
| *Medical recommendation* | Two recommendations: (a) medical practitioner with previous acquaintance of the patient; (b) medical practitioner specially approved by local health authority.<br>A joint recommendation (Form 3B) or separate recommendations made within seven days of each other are satisfactory (Form 3A). |
| *Grounds* | (a) Patient is suffering from mental disorder of a nature or degree which warrants detention for at least a limited period of observation. AND<br>(b) Is required for the patient's health or safety. OR<br>(c) Is required for the protection of other persons. |
| *Duration* | Not exceeding 28 days including day of admission. |
| *Renewal* | By an application under Section 26 (Treatment). |
| *Comments* | Each medical recommendation shall include a statement that the grounds of the application are complied with and must be signed on or before the date of the application.<br>One medical recommendation may be given by a doctor on the staff of the hospital admitting the patient (does not apply to nursing homes). It is often most appropriate for this to be the consultant who will subsequently treat the patient. |

## Section 26  Admission for treatment

| | |
|---|---|
| *Applicant* | (a)  Nearest relative (Form 4A) or (b)  Mental Welfare Officer (Form 4B) — Must have seen the patient within 14 days of date of application. |
| *Medical recommendation* | Two recommendations: (a) approved medical practitioner; (b) practitioner with previous acquaintance of the patient. A joint recommendation (Form 5B) or separate recommendations (Form 5A) are required. If separate examinations are made they must be within seven days of one another. |
| *Grounds* | (a)  Patient suffers from mental disorder (i)  Mental illness or severe subnormality. (ii)  If under 21 years of age, psychopathic disorder or subnormality and the disorder is of such a degree or nature to warrant detention in hospital for medical treatment AND (a)  Is required for the patient's health or safety OR (b)  Is required for the protection of other persons. |
| *Duration* | One year including the day of admission. |
| *Renewal* | From the end of the year mentioned above for a further year and then for periods of two years. It is the duty of the responsible medical officer (the consultant in charge of the case) to report to the managers of the hospital two months before expiration of each period. |

*Comment*

A Mental Welfare Officer must consult the nearest relative unless it would involve unreasonable delay or be impracticable. He may not make an application if the nearest relative objects.

If a psychopathic personality or a subnormal patient is also suffering from a mental illness he may be admitted under this section even if over the age of 21. The application must state his exact age if this is known or alternatively that he is believed to be under 21.

As with Section 25 one medical recommendation can be from a doctor on the staff of the admitting hospital.

## Section 29    Emergency admissions

| | | | |
|---|---|---|---|
| *Applicant* | (a) Any relative<br>or<br>(b) Mental Welfare Officer | Form 2 | Must see the patient within three days of application. |
| *Medical recommendation* | One recommendation (Form 3A) | | By practitioner having previous acquaintance with patient, if practicable.<br>Must see the patient on or before the date of application. |
| *Grounds* | (a) That admission for observation (as under Section 25) is urgently necessary.<br>AND<br>(b) That applying the procedure of Section 25 would occasion unreasonable delay. | | |
| *Duration* | Seventy-two hours (three days). | | |
| *Renewal* | By means of a second medical recommendation which must be signed and received by the hospital managers within the three days of emergency observation, i.e. Section 29 admission can thus be converted to Section 25 (Observation) or Section 26 (Treatment). | | |
| *Comments* | (i) No age limit for psychopathic personality or subnormality.<br>(ii) Recommendation should contain clinical evidence indicating why the case is urgent. | | |

## Section 30(2)   Patient already in hospital

| | |
|---|---|
| *Applicant* | (a) Nearest relative<br>  or<br>(b) Mental Welfare Officer } No form need be completed. |
| *Medical recommendation* | (i) Report from medical practitioner in charge of the patient that informal admission is no longer appropriate; this will normally be the consultant or in his absence the senior doctor for the time being having overall clinical responsibility for his patient.<br>(ii) Two medical recommendations complying with the provisions of Section 25 or Section 26.<br>*Note.* The patient may be detained for three days from (i) above, during which time application and two medical recommendations must be completed if longer detention is required. |
| *Grounds* | (i) Informal patient requires detention.<br>(ii) A period of treatment necessary following observation and patient unsuitable for informal status. |
| *Duration* | Three days. |
| *Renewal* | As for Section 25 or 26. |
| *Comments* | It is obvious that this procedure should be used as infrequently as possible since its free application would soon undermine the whole concept of treatment on an informal basis. |

## Section 33   Reception in guardianship

| | |
|---|---|
| *Applicant* | (a)  Nearest relative (Form 7A)<br>(b)  Mental Welfare Officer (Form 7B) |
| *Medical recommendation* | As for Section 26: (Form 8A) separate recommendations; (Form 8B) joint recommendations.<br>Patient must suffer from mental disorder as defined under Section 26 (including limitations in cases if psychopathy and subnormality) and<br>(a)  that the disorder is such as to warrant the patient's reception into guardianship;<br>(b)  that it is necessary in the patient's interests or for the protection of other persons. |
| *Duration* | As for Section 26. |
| *Renewal* | As for Section 26. |
| *Comments* | This section gives powers to control the place of residence and everyday life of the patient in the community. It has been likened to the control of a father over a child under the age of 14.<br>The person named as guardian may be the local health authority, but if not the application has no effect unless accepted by the local health authority. The application must be accompanied be a statement that the person named is willing to act as guardian. |

## PART IV   S 28

### Medical recommendations

Every application must be accompanied by two medical recommendations. One of these must be by a practitioner approved by the local health authority as having special experience in the diagnosis or treatment of mental disorders; and the other, if possible, by the patient's general practitioner.

## PART IV    S 36 and S 134 (Part IX)

### Correspondence of patients

Any letter addressed to a patient or written by a patient which would be calculated, in the opinion of the responsible medical officer or the guardian, to interfere with his treatment may be withheld and returned to the sender.

Letters addressed by a patient to any of the following may not be withheld: the Minister, any Member of Parliament, the Court of Protection, the managers of the hospital or the guardian, any other authority or person holding the power of discharge, a Mental Health Review Tribunal (if applicable) and a solicitor (if acting for the patient).

## PART IV    S 37–46

### Care, treatment and authority for detention

## PART IV    S 47

### Discharge of patients

The following authorities have power to discharge a patient who is compulsorily detained:

1    From S 29 (Emergency) patient is normally discharged after a lapse of 72 hours, unless S 29 is extended either to S 25 or to S 26.
2    From S 25 (Observation):
   (a)   The responsible medical officer;
   (b)   The managers of the hospital; and
   (c)   Automatically at the end of 28 days, unless S 25 is extended to S 26.
3    From S 26 (Treatment):
   (a)   The responsible medical officer;
   (b)   The managers of the hospitals;
   (c)   The nearest relative; and
   (d)   Automatically after one year, unless renewed.

## PART IV    S 48–59

### Relatives of patients and mental welfare officers

## PART V    S 60–80

### Hospital orders by the Courts
Compulsory admission to hospital or guardianship of mentally disordered persons convicted of offences by the Courts.

S 60    Written or oral evidence of two doctors that the offender is suffering from mental disorder warranting hospital treatment or guardianship; a particular hospital willing to receive him within 28 days; and this is the best method of dealing with him. *Note:* No age limit.

S 65    Designed to protect the public from mentally disordered offender convicted of a serious offence. Court of Assize or Quarter Sessions may order the admission of such a persistent offender to a hospital willing to receive him. Restriction is put on his discharge, leave or transfer, for which the consent of the Home Secretary is required. *Note:* Age 14 and over.

S 72    Transfer from penal establishments or approved schools.

## PART VI    S 81–96

### Removal and return of patients within the United Kingdom

## PART VII    S 97–99

### Special hospitals
Persons who require treatment under conditions of special security on account of their dangerous, violent or criminal propensities.

## PART VIII    S 100–121

### Management of property and affairs of patients

## PART IX   S 122–124

### Mental Health Review Tribunal

## PART IX   S 125–131

### Offences

Various offences against which action may be taken under the Act:
S 125   Forging with intent to deceive or wilfully making false entries in application for admission of patients to hospital or guardianship, medical recommendations, or any other relevant documents.

S 126   Ill-treatment of patients by an officer on the staff of a hospital.

S 127   The committing of sexual offences against mentally disordered patients.

S 128   Unlawful sexual intercourse on the part of an officer on the staff of a hospital with a woman patient.

S 129   Inducing or assisting a patient to become absent from a hospital, or knowingly harbouring such a patient.

S 130   Obstructing a person authorized under the Act to inspect any premises, to see the patient, to produce any document duly required, or to obstruct in any other way a person in the exercise of his functions.

S 131   Proceedings for any of these offences may be instituted by a local health authority.

## PART IX   S 135

### Neglect or ill-treatment

If a Mental Welfare Officer lays information on oath before a Justice of Peace of suspected ill-treatment or neglect of a mentally disordered person, a warrant authorizing his removal to a place of safety, for a period not exceeding 72 hours, may be issued. In the execution of the warrant, a constable shall be accompanied by a Mental Welfare Officer and a general practitioner to enter the premises.

A place of safety may be a residential accommodation provided by a local authority; a hospital or mental nursing home; a residential home for mentally disordered persons; a police station; and any other suitable place the occupier of which is willing to receive the patient.

## PART IX   S 136

### Found in a public place

A person who appears to be mentally disordered and in need of care or control, is in a place to which the public has access, he may be removed by a constable to a place of safety.

## PART IX   S 137

### Members of Parliament

Method of reporting to the speaker of the House of Commons about a Member of Parliament detained on grounds of mental disorder.

## PART IX   S 141

### Protection for Acts done in pursuance of this Act

No civil or criminal proceeding shall be brought against any person in any court, unless the act was done in bad faith or without reasonable care.

The proceedings can be instituted only by or with the consent of the Director of Public Prosecutions.

---

# Mental Health (Amendment) Act, 1975

Royal Assent: 8 May, 1975. Came into operation: 1 September, 1975.

---

An Act to enable potentially dangerous patients to be detained in institutions.